CIRCLES IN THE NURSERY:

Practicing Multicultural Family Therapy

Northern Virginia Family Service
Healthy Families - Alexandria
Help • Hope • Here
5249 Duke Street, Suite 308
Alexandria, VA 22304

CIRCLES IN THE NURSERY:

Practicing Multicultural Family Therapy

by Leena Banerjee Brown

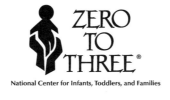

Washington, DC

Published by

ZERO TO THREE
2000 M St., NW, Suite 200, Washington, DC 20036-3307
(202) 638-1144; Toll-free orders (800) 899-4301
Fax: (202) 638-0851
Web: www.zerotothree.org

The mission of the ZERO TO THREE Press is to publish authoritative research, practical resources, and new ideas for those who work with and care about infants, toddlers, and their families. Books are selected for publication by an independent Editorial Board.

The views contained in this book are those of the authors and do not necessarily reflect those of ZERO TO THREE: National Center for Infants, Toddlers and Families, Inc.

These materials are intended for education and training to help promote a high standard of care by professionals. Use of these materials is voluntary and their use does not confer any professional credentials or qualification to take any registration, certification, board or licensure examination, and neither confers nor infers competency to perform any related professional functions.

The user of these materials is solely responsible for compliance with all local, state or federal rules, regulations or licensing requirements. Despite efforts to ensure that these materials are consistent with acceptable practices, they are not intended to be used as a compliance guide and are not intended to supplant or to be used as a substitute for or in contravention of any applicable local, state or federal rules, regulations or licensing requirements. ZERO TO THREE expressly disclaims any liability arising from use of these materials in contravention of such rules, regulations or licensing requirements.

The views expressed in these materials represent the opinions of the respective authors. Publication of these materials does not constitute an endorsement by ZERO TO THREE of any view expressed herein, and ZERO TO THREE expressly disclaims any liability arising from any inaccuracy or misstatement.

Cover design: Dan Pitts / e210.com

Text design and composition: K Art and Design, Inc.

Library of Congress Cataloging-in-Publication Data

Banerjee Brown, Leena.

    Circles in the nursery : practicing multicultural family therapy / by Leena Banerjee Brown.
       p. ; cm.
    ISBN 978-1-934019-09-2
    1. Family psychotherapy--Cross-cultural studies. 2. Psychiatry, Transcultural. I. Title.
    [DNLM: 1. Family Therapy--methods. 2. Child, Preschool. 3. Cultural Diversity. 4. Infant. WM 430.5.F2 B215c 2007]
    RC488.5.B334 2007
    616.89'156--dc22
                        2007014656

Copyright © 2007 by ZERO TO THREE. All rights reserved.

For permission for academic photocopying (for course packets, study materials, etc.) by copy centers, educators, or university bookstores or libraries, of this and other ZERO TO THREE materials, please contact Copyright Clearance Center, 222 Rosewood Drive, Danvers, MA 01923; phone (978) 750-8400; fax (978) 750-4744; or visit its Web site at www.copyright.com.

10 9 8 7 6 5 4 3 2 1

ISBN 978-1-934019-09-2

Printed in the United States of America

Suggested citation:
Banerjee Brown, L. (2007). *Circles in the nursery: Practicing multicultural family therapy.* Washington, DC: ZERO TO THREE.

DEDICATION

To my students—those journeying with me now, those who have in years past, and those who are to come. I am humbled by your courage to dive deeply into the experience and meanings of existence, to resurface enlivened, and to pass on the treasures of awareness to fellow beings—especially to the cycle of life embodied in infants, toddlers, young children, and their families.

TABLE OF CONTENTS

Preface xiii
Leena Banerjee Brown

PART I: CONCEPTUAL FRAMEWORK

Chapter 1
Presence in Multicultural Infant–Family Mental Health 3
Leena Banerjee Brown

Introduction 3

The Circles Framework 4
    Principle 1: Comprehensiveness 5
    Principle 2: Integration of Subjective and Objective Reality 6

Circles: Seven Circles of Awareness and Experience for Presence in Multicultural
Infant–Family Mental Health 8
    Circle One: Child Development and Sociocultural Identity Development 9
    Circle Two: Primary Caregiving Relationships 24
    Circle Three: Caregivers 27

References 30

Chapter 2
Family Systems and Culture 33
Leena Banerjee Brown

Circle Four: Family Systems and Culture, An Introduction 33

Structural Family Therapy 38
    Structural Questions: Suggestions for Clinicians 43

Strategic Family Therapy 44
    Strategic Questions: Suggestions for Clinicians 50

Paradoxical Family Therapy 50
    Paradoxical Questions: Suggestions for Clinicians 53

Bowenian Family Therapy 54
    Bowenian Questions: Suggestions for Clinicians 57

Conclusion 57

References 59

Chapter 3
Self-Awareness, Presence, and the Growth of Presence 61
Leena Banerjee Brown

Circle Five: Self-Awareness: Clinician's Reflective Narratives 61

Circle Six: Clinician Presence in the Holding of Relationships (Interpersonal World) 71

Circle Seven: Creating Sustaining Space: Personally–Culturally Meaningful Self-Care, Generating Presence (Simultaneous Access to Intrapersonal and Interpersonal Worlds) 76

References 79

PART II: CHRONICLES OF CLINICAL CASE APPLICATIONS

Chapter 4
Kevin's Early Infancy: Regulation and Well-Being Through Innovations in Multicultural Infant–Family Mental Health 83
Leena Banerjee Brown

Introduction 83
    Presenting Problem 84
    Family and Placement History 84
    Mental Health Interventions and Outcomes 85

Kevin's Case and the Circles Framework 89

Research Bases That Assisted Me in My Work With Kevin: Hidden and Unhidden Trauma in Infancy and Early Childhood 91

    Innovative Interventions: Touch, Regulation, and Well-Being 95

    Innovative Interventions: Sound, Regulation, and Well-Being 96

Questions 98

References 99

Chapter 5
Identity and Difference: Mark "and I Don't Like That Brown" 101
Leena Banerjee Brown

Introduction 101

Relevant History 102

Needs and Strengths. 103

Therapeutic Process: Observations, Interventions, and Outcomes 105
    Phase I 105
    Phase II 107
    Phase III 109

Reflections Using the Circles Framework 112
    Circle One: Development 112
    Circle Two: Caregiving Relationships 113
    Circle Three: Primary Caregiver 114
    Circle Four: Family Relationships 114
    Circle Five: Clinician's Reflections 117
    Circle Six: Clinician Presence 117
    Circle Seven: Self-Care 119

Questions 119

Chapter 6
A Time to Follow and a Time to Lead: Feeling "At-Home" With Circles 121
Lucia Lopez-Plunkett and Leena Banerjee Brown

Introduction 121

Circle One: "He Chooses Not to Listen!" 122

Circle Two: "I Think the Asthma Medication Makes Him Excited." 123

Circle Three: "But I Am Calm!". 127

Circle Four: "If the Family Had a Voice, What Would It Say?" 128

Circle Five: "Can You Be My Other Grandson's Therapist?" 128

Circle Six: "Am I Being Authentic?" 130

Circle Seven: "Are My Feelings Really That Heavy?" 132

References 134

PART III: PROGRAM AND RESEARCH APPLICATIONS

Chapter 7
Thriving in the Clinic: Reflections on Early Connections, a Multicultural Infant–Family Community Mental Health Program 137
Matthew Calkins, Leena Banerjee Brown, and Michael Barraza

Introduction 137

The Early Connections Population: Reflections on Overburdened Families and Overburdened Systems 138

A "Good Enough" Provider: The Precursors of Early Connections 139

Movement Through Grief to Hope: Using Process and Context to Begin Program Development 140

Renewal: The Birth of Early Connections 141

Foundations: Training and Circles 143

Collaborations: Opportunities for Growth 146

Reflections on Leadership 150

Balance: Final Reflections 151

References 152

Chapter 8
Early Connections Process Research and Circles: Presence in the Training Experience and New Horizons in Research 153
Rajeswari Natrajan, Leena Banerjee Brown, Tasha Boucher, Matthew Calkins, Lucia Lopez-Plunkett, Brooke Nisen, and Patricia Rosas

The Circles Training Model 155

Setting of the Circles Training 156

Methodology 156
    Participants 157
    Data Collection 158
    Establishing Credibility and Authenticity of the Study 159

Data Analysis 161

Results and Discussion 161
    How Did Participants Learn? 162
    What Did Participants Learn? Themes Regarding Therapeutic Presence . . . 173

Conclusion 177

References 180

EPILOGUE

Chapter 9
The Placental Ground of Experience—A Source of Connection, Meaning, and Presence: Paradigmatic Considerations 185
Leena Banerjee Brown

References 191

About the Authors 193

PREFACE

In *Circles*, I have put together a conceptual approach that is simultaneously inward and outward in its focus and integrates knowledge from various fields. These fields include human development, psychotherapy, family systems, multicultural psychology, and process research as they integrate and come together for work in multicultural infant–family mental health. The approach is in-depth, multidimensional, and comprehensive. The elements in *Circles* are ones that I have used routinely in my own grassroots-level work in communities in Hawaii and Southern California through community mental health programs. These elements have helped me connect with and effectively respond to the needs of babies and families in conditions of poverty, marginalization, and stigmatization, and their natural impulses to cope, thrive, and grow, and to the potential in communities and society to change and grow from the ground up. At the same time, this approach has kept me connected and attentive to my own instincts, needs, and growth and has helped me create necessary balances in my life that have energized each new day and challenge and have enabled me to face them with humility, hope, and ingenuity. On the basis of this experience I have written *Circles* as an invitation to those who work with the human nursery, to consider the process route to self knowledge, epistemology, theory, practice, and research.

Among the many fortunate events that have occurred in the writing of *Circles*, one was the enthusiastic interest that the Early Connections program showed in adopting the Circles framework in its training. This interest led to a 9-month phase of training in self-awareness development (Circle Five activities) and self-care practices (Circle Seven activities), along with ongoing reflective supervision and an accompanying research study on these complex training processes. We were able to use a brilliant process methodology called the *significant moments methodology*, which was used by child–family clinician researchers at the Tavistock Clinics in the United Kingdom. Our process researcher came to the program in the most organic and timely way imaginable, and the energy, relationships, and work in the group facilitated an aliveness and agency that we call presence—a characteristic that clinicians can take their whole careers to achieve. As a result of this combined collective training and research endeavor, the Circles framework was transformed into a live model in which Circle Five and Circle Seven training led clinicians to actively take inward and outward journeys more deeply and thoroughly in working with all aspects of cases and with the subject matter of the content-rich circles (i.e., Circles One through Four). The third section of this book documents and illustrates this work for replication and technical assistance to other multicultural infant–family programs around the country and the globe.

Presence (Circle Six) is a focal point of *Circles* created by integrating the technical information of Circles One through Four with the self-awareness development of Circle Five. This presence is continually regenerated by investment in Circle Seven. In other words, technical content, skills, and self-awareness flow through the aliveness of one's presence into one's interactions in work and in life and are sustained through attuned self-care practices. The exploration of presence in Early Connections training and research has revealed its deeper core as a multilayered process that connects multiple levels of self and experience in the world. Being present means being here—in the flesh, in present time, and attentive to the present moment. It means being open, available, and responsive to empathic connection and relationships with others. It means having connection and access to the unbounded, creative, and ubiquitous within and without. Through being present ourselves, we give all that is needed and all that we can in our roles as clinicians, program developers, organizational stakeholders, policymakers, and, indeed, authors working together to make real the foundational work of enhancing and enriching the lives of babies, families, and societies.

There are several overarching areas in which *Circles* offers contributions. The first is in family systems by (a) encouraging the inclusion of whole family systems as well as extended family and community systems in multicultural infant–family mental health and (b) providing the tools of family systems therapy to do so. This approach extends the robust dyadic approaches in the field for inclusion of the family relationships in which dyads are, invariably, nested. In fact, an important insight from the study of family systems has been that the smallest natural unit in relationship systems is a triad and not a dyad, as dyads regularly become triads for purposes of navigating stress and stabilizing themselves. A family systems approach is also more consistent and resonant with the world views of people in many cultures, particularly nondominant people, such as people of color, in this country and around the world. *Circles* offers knowledge and tools for conceptualizing, strategizing, and, most important, engaging and being in relationships with families of diverse cultures to help them and their babies enjoy a fuller life.

Diversity is an overarching area of contribution in *Circles*. Its importance in current and future societies cannot be overstated, yet we are slow to face up to it and own it. Diversity continually challenges the comfort of the familiar and the known and calls to our daring to meet new horizons of openness and new depths of compassion. How can we prepare ourselves to meet the task of helping the Hispanic American parents of Kevin (in chapter 4), the 3-month-old African American boy who had a lucky landing with a third set of parents in his third month of life, consistently communicate to him his value as an African American male child in this society and in this world? How do we empower

Carlos' (chapter 6) parenting grandparents to facilitate his positive identification with unique aspects of his mixed heritage identity? How do we empower the embattled yet courageous Caucasian American father of Mark (chapter 5), who entrusts his children to the care of Hispanic American caregivers and passes on to them his unconscious, denigrating attitudes toward people of color? How do we help him deal effectively with the anguish, anger, and ambivalence that this behavior leaves Mark with in emotionally meaningful relationships with people of color? How do we work with the intergenerationally transmitted unpreparedness that the family has, as a whole, in engaging openly, positively, and comfortably with diversity? The challenges in Mark's family are shared widely in the human family, yet diversity is a challenge from which we can no longer hide. A scan of demographics in our society and technology-facilitated interconnectedness of the global community signal that diversity is a phenomenon whose time has come. *Circles* offers a way to make contact with diversity through exploration of lived experiences, genuine and reliable peer relationships that support this exploration, and guidance from the literature and mentors. *Circles* uses the term *multicultural infant–family mental health* to encourage the idea that diversity is a part and parcel of the fabric and substance of the field and not a special consideration or topic within it.

Process research methodology is a further area of contribution by *Circles*. This methodology facilitates the study of the complexities of process that occur in the clinical encounter as well as in human interactions in general. Process research is an encompassing and flexible methodology that can adapt to the natural state and natural environment of the phenomenon being studied, thus capturing the fullness, complexity, and meaning of lived experiences. Both qualitative and quantitative studies can be conducted through process research. *Circles* reports on the first of four cycles of qualitative data on training research and reflective supervision in multicultural infant–family mental health. A subsequent project now underway is collecting quantitative data. Process research is a research approach with interdisciplinary methodologies developed in the fields of family systems therapy, counseling psychology, and anthropology, among others. It is an important approach that can answer—in sensitive and thorough ways—numerous questions in multicultural infant–family mental health. Such use of process research will develop a knowledge base that is rich and applicable. It will also pioneer the broadening of the definition of evidence in useful ways, as good evidence and outcomes are invariably dependent on good process.

Circles is, ultimately, about being at home in oneself—in one's family, work, community, and the world. It is about going where each of us can go within ourselves—to infancy, an experience we can share despite the varieties of our lives. I grew up in India, an old and fertile land where the earth, wind, and rain whisper the wisdoms of the ages, if we care to hear. It is a land where the ancients sat around fires and created voluminous, orally transmitted texts of metaphysical, lyrical prose and poetry called the Vedas and Upanishads. These works, originally in Sanskrit, speak with a purity and clarity that can reach beyond words to the infant in each of our experience and to our capacity for nonconceptual, experiential knowing. This capacity for the simple, true joy of connecting and knowing beyond words is a capacity that helps us in our work in multicultural infant–family mental health because it takes us to this nonverbal horizon with parents, families, and their preverbal babies. *Circles* offers a pathway for being grounded and free (in the words of the Early Connections lead researcher) on this horizon through the finding, re-finding, and cultivating of ordinary, daily opportunities to do so. Sometimes, we need not only to turn our attention to what is and has been around us but to look and hear with new interest and awareness. I share an example, a poem, from my own family of the moving connectedness between a teenage boy observing and enjoying the natural process of his 2-year-old sister's play.

> *Lost to the world, little Jhunu at play,*
> *While I watch her in silence this day,*
> *She needs but little—no elaborate toy,*
> *A sheet and a shawl bring so much joy,*
> *Small things like these can go miles,*
> *To keep little Jhunu radiant in smiles.*

—Lt. General Ashish Banerjee, PVSM (Retd.)
written in 1946, in Patna, India,
translated from Bengali into English in 2006

The poet is my father at 13 years of age, taking a deep, affectionate, and creative interest in his youngest sister's play. Such simple moments of shared joy and meaning last a lifetime and build capacity—both neural and experiential—for empathy, relationship, and presence.

Circles was written by the confluence of grace and generosity of sources so numerous that I cannot name them all. From the depths of my being, I thank each and every person who has helped me, and I name but a few who I cannot leave unnamed. Emily Fenichel, my first editor, and the ZERO TO THREE Press lit the spark within me to write *Circles*. Emily's encouragement and vision that these *Circles* carry the scope of Bronfenbrenner's work of 30 years ago, but in different ways, has stayed with me after her passing and has influenced this work. The team at the ZERO TO THREE Press has been a source of consistent and stellar professional support. My family (across continents) has been a constant source of love and support. My peers at the university (across institutions, and particularly at Alliant International University, California School of Professional Psychology, Los Angeles) have been a source of vital collegial connection, and my colleagues in community mental health (across institutions, and particularly at Early Connections) have been an equally vital source of inspiration. The gift of time from Alliant International University has been valuable in facilitating the completion of this book.

In closing, I bow to the light in the void, the universal cradle from whence I come, in words that are first cited in Sanskrit and then translated into English:

Twameva Mata, cha pita twameva,
Twameva bandhu, shakha twameva,
Twameva vidya, dravinam twameva,
Twameva sarvam, mama deva deva.
Om Shanti, Om Shanti, Om Shanti.

Thou art my mother, thou art my father,
Thou art my friend, thou art my companion,
Thou art knowledge, thou art wealth,
Thou art all in all, oh Lord!
Om peace, Om peace, Om peace.

PART I: CONCEPTUAL FRAMEWORK

CHAPTER 1

Presence in Multicultural Infant–Family Mental Health

Leena Banerjee Brown

Awareness is realization. It is integrating all aspects of experience to advance insight and well-being that are a means to thriving.

> *The art of life has an impudence; it will not be observed, it has to be experienced from within.*
> —Ralph Waldo Emerson

Experience is a container in which awareness is born. Connections/relationships, perceptions, actions, feelings, thoughts, and memories, and all possible combinations of these, create our continuous stream of experiences, be they in conscious awareness or not. They also create discontinuous leaps in our experience, giving us deep and expansive, intuitive insight.

Introduction

To enter the life of an infant or young child and to share in the experience of this child's family is to have the privilege of participating at the beginning of life and at the beginning of a cycle of family life.[1] It is in this foundational, formative time that our work in multicultural infant–family mental health occurs. This work calls for an increasingly informed, sophisticated, and subtle integration of knowledge and experience that flows with our uniquely human capacities for empathy and intuition.

---

[1] The author gratefully acknowledges the valuable editorial work given to *Circles* by Rudra Amadeus B. B. (Rudy) Roy.

The goal of this book is to advance the capacity of the professional to be present to see, hear, and engage with the infant's and young child's subtle and varied communications as well as with those individuals in its nexus of culturally meaningful caregiving and family relationships.

We know from classic and ongoing interdisciplinary studies that relationships provide the crucial context for the development and well-being of infants and young children. The key component in these relationships is human connection, the reliable, warm, and understanding presence of an adult articulated in the literature as attunement and attachment. Correspondingly, in professional relationships in multicultural infant–family mental health such as in the client–professional relationship and in intra- and interagency collegial collaborations, few capacities are more crucial than the capacities for connection and empathy. Increasing awareness by increasing the practice of reflecting on and integrating all aspects of experience facilitates deeper, more complex understandings of relationships in their cultural contexts. Such practice increases a professional's capacity for connecting and being present in relationships. In this way, awareness gained from experience enhances and advances the capacity for presence—being alive in the moment, connected to self and to others.

The Circles Framework

Thus, *Circles* offers a framework that focuses on building multicultural infant–family mental health professionals' capacities for presence in the clinical domain. These capacities can be put to equally good use in other domains of multicultural infant–family mental health such as program development, research, or policy. The Circles framework is built on two principles: (a) comprehensiveness and (b) integration of the subjective and objective information. It is also built on my experience of 20 years working at the front lines of community mental health and my attention to the contributions of my own culture and immigrant status to my professional identity, multicultural infant–family work, and rearing of three children. My multicultural infant–family work following my doctoral training started with development of the tertiary prevention part of Healthy Start (Clinton, 1996) in Hawaii called Mother–Infant Support Team (MIST). In this program, we worked at the cusp of prevention and treatment, connecting with infants, their parents, and families at birth, when an older sibling in the family had had a case history with Child Protective Services. The Imminent and Threatened Harm arm of the law in Hawaii facilitated such proactive engagement. MIST provided psychosocial and developmental assessment, home visiting, nursing support, parenting groups, parent support groups, and family therapy services. Native Hawaiian families, the most disenfranchised group on the island, were overrepresented in the population served. Many innovations were needed for effective outreach to this group beyond their legitimate, intergenerationally established fears of outsiders. Notable among these outreach efforts was my experience of going out to remote north shore Native

Hawaiian family homesteads with experienced, local program staff to "talk story" and build connection in respectful and organic ways. The outcomes tracked by the program recorded improvements in the quality of parent–child interaction and reduction of Child Protective Service reports in target families. In addition, risk factors were reduced through increased parental connection with children facilitated by improved parenting skills, increased awareness of early development, and improved access to community resources (Banerjee, 1989, 1990).

My work with families and young children continued in community mental health in Los Angeles County, California, through services such as psychological and developmental testing, dyadic and family therapy, program development, and reflective supervision. Graduate teaching, training, and applied and secondary research supervision of clinical psychology doctoral students occurred in parallel at Alliant International University's California School of Professional Psychology. In this training, multicultural psychology and community clinical psychology were integrated with family systems therapy for young children in families. This work at the university continues today. In the past 2 years, I have been a part of creating and developing a new outpatient community mental health program called Early Connections at Bienvenidos Children's Center. In this program, which is discussed in Part III of this book, the staff members are actively working with the Circles framework.

Principle 1: Comprehensiveness

The first principle of comprehensiveness involves the use of a broad contextual lens that includes the infant and young child and the reciprocal relationships with caregivers, with family and community, and with the multicultural infant mental health professional. Family systems theory and practice have amply demonstrated that triangles are the basic building blocks of families (Guerin, Fogarty, Fay, & Kautto, 1996). Dyads are inherently unstable, so they routinely and predictably recruit third members to cope with dyadic stress. In this way, dyads flexibly shift into triads, defuse anxiety, and return to dyadic states of stability. Flexible, interlocking triangles constitute building blocks of healthy relational/family systems. Thus, this principle of comprehensiveness encourages the multicultural infant mental health professional to take at least a triadic relational perspective embedded in family and community systems. It calls for genuine engagement with sociocultural contexts in which people reside and which infants inherit. It calls for awareness and understanding of the sociohistorical and sociopolitical realities of these sociocultural contexts that affect everyday experience. It calls for interdisciplinary collaboration in data gathering and synthesis of complex data covering a multiplicity of interactions. The holding of this complex information with presence and clarity provides the professional with a coherent picture of a whole data set from which new, relevant, and respectful insights can emerge. At the same time, the framework is amenable to a focus on any subset of its canvas, should this be salient or necessary to do at a particular point in time.

Principle 2: Integration of Subjective and Objective Reality

The second principle involves the integration of subjective and objective information in the ground of experience. To do this, Circles uses Bowen's (1985) juxtaposition of intrapersonal and interpersonal realms of experience. Alternating intrapersonal and interpersonal circles are used for experiencing and understanding the world of the infant/young child and family. In both realms, scientific information on relevant psychological, developmental, social, biological, and cultural factors is considered, in addition to subjective, experiential aspects of these realms, resulting in an integrated, deeply attentive understanding of the phenomena at hand. Thus the clinician asks herself, "What is my experience internally and relationally across circles in this case, how does this relate to the information from assessments, observations, and the literature, and how do I integrate the two usefully to help my clients?" In taking this approach, Circles is merely highlighting an important component that is routinely used in clinical work but is insufficiently owned in professional psychological/mental health paradigms. This approach does not present something entirely new. Rather, it says that this invisible but palpable experiential aspect of the work in multicultural infant mental health is of vital importance both for knowledge bases and applications of it. This approach also says that it is empowering for the field if it owns and integrates subjective experience with traditionally derived empirical data in the scientific foundations of knowledge as a component that is not only valid but indispensable.

Assessment, intervention, and research in the field already include relationship building, interviewing, observing, using narrow-band or broadband scales, interventions informed by evidence and self-report. In each of these activities, the subjective participation of the professional produces subtle but detectable variations. Underlying all of these activities is experience, the container in which subjective and objective information and conscious and unconscious information is integrated. Experience is the container in which connection occurs between what is inside oneself (sensations, feelings, thoughts, memories) and what is outside oneself (people, relationships, bodies of knowledge). In this container of experience, we proceed individually and collectively in states that are coherent or incoherent, fractured or whole to engage in various types of decision-making processes. These processes in the field of multicultural infant–family mental health have to do with the development and well-being of young children and the contexts (caregiving relationships, families, and communities) that hold them.

Our quest for knowledge continues to be guided by a paradigm that treats subjective aspects of experience as impurities that we need to filter out to provide the clear and objective view of phenomenon. As a result systematic, rigorous, and varied means of accessing and using subjectively elicited information remains largely outside our professional dialogue and professional methodologies. This leaves our understanding of the dedication, discipline, and methods of introspection and deep reflection, all of which are necessary for reaching clarity and useful knowledge through subjective processes, greatly undeveloped in our allied fields. Further, as is common with that which is not well-understood, the subjective route to knowledge is devalued and subjugated to the objective route. Yet the significance of subjective experience cannot be overstated in a field in which connection and empathic understanding open the door, for the professional, to the early worlds of the infant and caregiver across relationships, families, and communities. The absence of rigorous attention to the subjective creates a loss and a gap in the field. Bridging this gap can engender support for fuller, more vital, and more humane professional engagement and training models in the multicultural infant–family field.

This principle of integrating the subjective and objective aspects of knowing is a call for holding, integrating, and moving beyond the dialectical tensions between the art and science of multicultural infant–family mental health into an integrated science. It is a call for clinicians to claim the opportunity that comes with each new birth and cycle of family life and to renew our hope for integrated development of knowledge in our futures. This second principle is a hope for a pathway to healing our fractured connections within (e.g., in ourselves), which is revealed in fractured connections without (e.g., in hierarchical relationships between domains of knowledge, methodologies for gaining knowledge, cultures in the human family, humans, and nature). The second principle is also about the hope for developing our natural human capacities to know and to thrive and for using these capacities toward the well-being and thriving of new generations of infants and young children.

Self-awareness development is a route that can contribute to a comprehensive and integrated approach to multicultural infant–family mental health. It includes the use of reflective practices in supervision (Heffron, 2005; Shahmoon-Shanok, Gilkerson, Eggbeer, & Fenichel, 1995) and in peer and collegial interactions as well as the use of parallel process/flow/mind (Csikszentmihalyi, 1990; Siegal, 1999). Self-awareness places a premium on commitment and active responsibility for personal development and well-being (self-care–based growth) in relationships, including collegial relationships, and on creating institutional environments (Shahmoon-Shanok, Lapidus, Grant, Halpern, & Lamb-Parker, 2005) that support these values and practices. Essentially, individuals, groups, and institutions that invest in self-awareness development undertake the privilege and the responsibility of work in multicultural infant–family mental health by putting themselves on an equal plane with those with whom they work. The process of engaging in learning through getting in touch with one's own story and process—and becoming comfortable with sharing, exploring, and expanding it for the purpose of professional development—calls for comfort with vulnerability. It takes the mask off of professionalism—that is, the professional persona—and encourages more humane, authentic presence and interactions in the workplace. It requires and inspires higher levels of collegial integrity and maturity for creating and sustaining work environments of transparency, honesty, and humility that put each person on the same level with others. It makes collaboration a reality because collaboration in multicultural infant–family practice grows out of living, creating, and being supported by a culture of collaboration in the organizations/institutions through which the work is done. Thus, self-awareness development emphasizes and encourages, first and foremost, our humanity as professionals.

Presence, or aliveness and connectedness in the present moment, is facilitated by the two principles of comprehensiveness and integration of subjective and objective reality. The former facilitates openness and expansiveness, and the latter facilitates integration, clarity, and coherence. Together, they prepare the multicultural infant–family mental health clinician to be aware, attuned, and present in holding complex, comprehensive information in complex, interrelated relationships.

Circles: Seven Circles of Awareness and Experience for Presence in Multicultural Infant–Family Mental Health

This book offers seven circles as a way of organizing its framework. The first four circles emphasize comprehensive technical information (objective information). The fifth circle introduces systematic self-awareness information (subjective information). Circle Six, which is the heart of the Circles framework, encourages integration of the information from all previous circles, so that the objective and subjective information flows through the presence of the professional in the moment. Circle Seven speaks to the need for self-care and for organizational contexts that sustain and support the growth of such presence. More specifically, these circles are as follows:

- The circle of the intrapersonal world of the child (Circle One: Child's Development, Nutrition, and Sociocultural Identity);

- The interpersonal world of the child and caregiver (Circle Two: Caregiving Relationship(s), Attunement, Attachment, and Culture);

- The intrapersonal world of the caregiver (Circle Three: Care-Receiving History, Caregiver Mental Health History, Caregiver States of Mind, and Culturally Influenced Developmental and Socialization Expectations and Practices);

- The interpersonal world of the child and caregivers' family and culture (Circle Four: Family Structure, Patterns, Supports, Sociohistorical Context, Sociopolitical Context, Cultural Resources, Cultural Traditions, Routines, and Rhythms);

- The intrapersonal world of the professional (Circle Five: Reflections on Personal History, Resources, Barriers, and Countertransference);

- The interpersonal world of the therapeutic relationship and presence (Circle Six: Interpersonal Holding of Child, Parents, and Family in Cultural Context [constituting clinical presence and the parallel process of holding in reflective supervision]); and

- The simultaneously intrapersonal and interpersonal circle of awareness (Circle Seven: Creating Sustaining Spaces From Which to Generate Personally and Culturally Attuned Self-Care That Feeds and Builds Presence).

This first chapter will deal with Circles One through Three, the second chapter will address Circle Four, and the third chapter will complete the discussion on Circles Five through Seven.

The field of multicultural infant mental health has well-developed repositories of knowledge and practice strategies in the areas of child development, primary caregiver–child relationship, and primary caregiver(s), which are covered in the first three circles. Therefore, these areas will merely be mentioned rather than covered in detail, with the exception of a section on sociocultural identity in Circle One. This approach is based on the assumption that readers are not only well-acquainted with these circles but have numerous ideas, experiences, and research evidence that supports their work with these circles. The Circles framework is built on the assumption that professionals will use that which they are already using and finding helpful and will integrate into it that which is new and relevant in this framework. (See Figure 1.1.)

Circle One: Child Development and Sociocultural Identity Development

Child development has benefited from the investment of thinkers, observers, practitioners, and researchers across several fields and offers the multicultural infant mental health professional an array of information and guidance on physical, nutritional, neural, psychomotor, socioemotional, and cognitive aspects of development. Information on developmental milestones and temperament, observation of infants and young children across multiple contexts, use of quick and/or comprehensive screens of developmental functioning, observation of parent–child interaction across contexts, and parent interviews are in the routine repertoire of the multicultural infant–family mental health professional.

The enormous energies invested over the past decade or more by professionals in multicultural infant–family mental health such as Stanley Greenspan (e.g., Greenspan & Benderly, 1997; Greenspan & Weider, 1998) and Bruce Perry (2003), and those such as Daniel Goleman (1995) addressing a wider audience have successfully shown that socioemotional development is primary to overall development and well-being and that it interplays critically with cognitive development, adjustment, and success in the world. Tools such as the Functional Emotional Assessment Scale (FEAS; Greenspan, DeGangi, & Weider, 2001) make complex understandings of the process of socioemotional development in the early years available for use. Using the FEAS, observing the developmental progression of achieving attentive, calm internal states; beginning the process of connecting in relationships; establishing reciprocal communications in these relationships; connecting feelings and

Figure 1.1 Circles: Seven circles of awareness and experience for presence in multicultural infant–family mental health.[2]

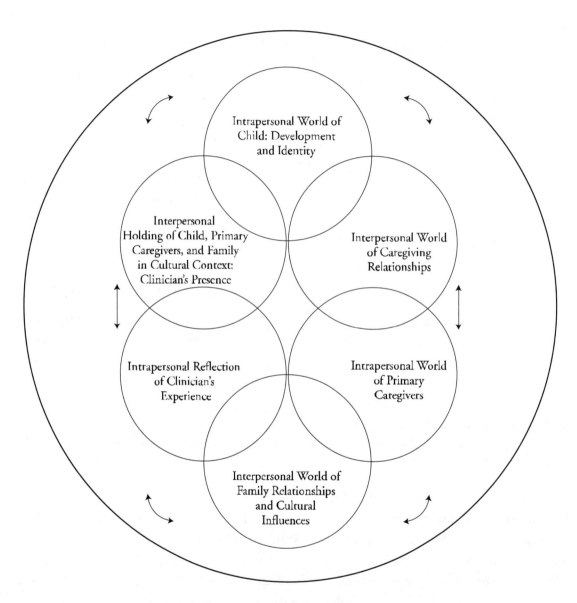

Intrapersonal and interpersonal awareness: Alive to connection and process

---

[2] We gratefully acknowledge the generosity and creativity of Matt and Kate Calkins in computerizing this graphic representation of Circles.

ideas and expressing them; and expressing more elaborate emotional ideas and more complex emotional thinking are invaluable ways of grasping and working with these complex, interconnected processes.

My clinical experience with this scale suggests that the first stage can be further differentiated into two stages—first, direct intrapersonal connection to sensory and emotional experiences within the skin that include calm, alert states and that give rise to the earliest self feelings, followed by the experience of interpersonal or dyadic regulation and achievement of quiet, calm, attentive, alert states. In other words, the infant may feel happy, comfortable, and content; he may feel too much sound, heat, and cold; or he may become hungry, get disquieted and fussy, and cry. These are some of the first connections with intrapersonal experience within the skin at the levels of physiology, sensation, emotion, and being. The infant senses, feels, and expresses this existential experience of being and, therefore, is. The primary caregiver's emotional availability to attend, sensitivity to accurately read, and responsivity to meet the infant's needs sets up patterns of early regulation of sensory and emotional experience. Through these experiences of regulation, the infant bridges experiences of equilibrium and disequilibrium to achieve calm, alert states more reliably and begins to develop the capacity to attend to the world.

The infant's affinity for the sound and touch of the primary caregiver occurs from the early days and weeks of life and has survival value. Erikson's (1963) work adds social–contextual meaning to the infant self within the skin and its early regulation:

The first demonstration of social trust in the baby is the ease of his feeding, the depth of his sleep, the relaxation of his bowels. The experience of mutual regulation of his increasingly receptive capacities with the maternal techniques of provision gradually helps him to balance the discomfort caused by the immaturity of homeostasis with which he was born. In his gradually increasing waking hours he finds that more and more adventures of the senses arouse a feeling of familiarity, of having coincided with a feeling of inner goodness (p. 247).

Repeated experiences of reliable, attuned care and feelings of inner calm, goodness, and well-being contribute to a psychological sense of trust in the world, of one's apparatus in the world, and of one's trustworthiness in relationships in the world. They help the infant in the first year of life to constructively resolve the dilemma of trust versus distrust. These experiences are the early basis of motivation and hope (Erikson, 1963). Progressive experiences of connection and regulation along with muscular maturation prepare the toddler for the second psychosocial task of autonomy versus doubt and shame. Exploration of the environment comes naturally with the capacity for greater mobility. The way in which this natural urge is guided by caregivers depends on the set of meanings (or culture) by which they are influenced. Keeping a more active young child safe may be a universal component of caregiving intention and behavior, whereas the extent and meaning attributed to exploration may vary widely among cultures, subcultures, and, indeed, family cultures. Not only is there no one way to do healthy child rearing, but there are so very many ways that come from the diversities of our experience as a species that it can readily boggle our minds as professionals. Childproofing a home and taking great joy and pride in a toddler's unceasing curiosities, mobility, and exploration may be a snapshot of a familial–cultural context for one child at this stage. Graduating an infant from what one might call the "held children" phase (held in the warmth of caregiving arms) to toddlerhood, in which Mead (1935) described them as "knee children" (p. 40) and, later, as "yard children" (p. 41), may be the familial–cultural context of another child at this stage. Repeated experiences of oneself as a separate acting person in the world kept safe by reliable and attuned caregivers with predictable rules that fit the cultural context are the basis of early self-control and willpower (Erikson, 1963). As the toddler and young child moves on to the task of initiative versus guilt, he continues to build more relationships in the family and with peers. He learns to explore and act upon the world in expanding ways, recover from distress with the help of caregiving relationships, and identify with the same-sex parent. Through these experiences, the child develops the early basis for direction and purpose in the world (Erikson, 1963).

Circle One is an opportunity for multicultural infant–family mental health professionals to consider and prepare, in a connected and regulated way, to work with the developmental tasks of connection, regulation, and communication in infancy and early childhood. Regulation itself traverses a developmental passage from interpersonal/dyadic regulation or guided regulation (Sroufe, Egeland, Carlson, & Collins, 2005) to self-regulation. Attention to parallel internal and interpersonal processes offers opportunities for refining professional and personal awareness, thus creating possibilities for experiencing deeper attunement, empathy, and insights relevant to a range of purposes in the work.

Sociocultural Identity: Connection to Self in Context and Multiple Layers of Identity

Sociocultural identity is a part of socioemotional development and refers to the infant and young child's emerging sense of themselves in their skin, in their caregiving relationships, and in their experiential world. There has been a focus on identity in adolescence since Erikson (1963) proposed that human beings struggle with the task of defining their identity in the world versus struggling with identity confusion or diffusion. However, not all children in the world experience adolescence, which is a cultural construction, and questions of identity are now being considered as occurring earlier in childhood. We are living in a society created by more than 2 centuries of immigration. Social policies of oppressive cultural homogenization, constructed to deal with the immense cultural diversity of the polity, have gradually given way to an active struggle to make sense of pluralism through the ideology and practices of multiculturalism (Banerjee, 2002). In addition, the world is becoming a smaller global village, and our economic, political, and, if we wake up to it, socioemotional futures are inextricably tied together. Migration is becoming a phenomenon that includes global mobility as well as immigration. The multicultural paradigm also is evolving from focusing on separate but equal cultures to seeking reasonable means of cohesion between cultures as well as maintaining the dynamic tensions and richness of different but equal cultures (Banerjee, 2002). The current focus on multiple layers of identity is an exemplification of this paradigm, as it encourages us to look at ourselves in complex ways, socialize our children in complex ways, and experience common ground with every other person because each person has multiple, complex layers of identity that affect their lives. The shift in language in multicultural writing from (until half a decade ago) dominant and oppressed cultures to (more recently) macro- and microcultures (Day & Parlakian, 2003) also is indicative of a multicultural paradigm that is not fighting for its existence in the social fabric but, rather, is speaking for growth and refinement in awareness.

In current times and in our foreseeable futures, infants and young children will be exposed to diversity in themselves and in their social contexts in an unprecedented way. Their parents, families, and communities will have the opportunities to help them make meaning of this diversity and cope with this complexity with resilience and hope. A longitudinal study of immigration points to two important, inevitable challenges in a global world—the presence of difference and of complexity (Suarez-Orozco & Qin-Hilliard, 2004). An approach to thriving in the nursery in such a global world must include resilient attitudes and practices toward difference and complexity. What better starting place than the puzzling intricacies at the core of socioemotional identity? Is this not a seat of self-determination, be it at a species, community, family, dyad, or individual level?

Architecture of Emerging Sociocultural Identity in Infants and Young Children

Clinical insight, scholarship, and research are brought together to create and offer a conceptualization of the architecture of an infant and young child's emerging sociocultural identity through the use of five elements. These elements are presented in a developmental progression from perceptual–motor and socioemotional development in the first triad to an integration of these developmental aspects with cognitive development in the later dyad.

The socioemotional triad consists of the following elements:

- Element 1: Connection to self. The experience of connection with sensations/perceptions and feelings within one's skin, the earliest experiences of presence or of simply being.

- Element 2: Dyadic regulation of self. The experience in primary caregiving relationships that makes it possible for the infant and young child to be calm and to attend, to experience continuity of self within the skin, despite periodic intensity of sensations/perceptions and feelings in response to events and needs.

- Element 3: Self in relational context. The experience of connection to self in caregiving relationships, which when attuned to the infant, facilitate internal working models of security (Bowlby, 1953, 1969, 1973, 1980), trust (Erikson, 1963), engagement, and reciprocity (Greenspan & Benderly, 1997) and healthy self-feelings consisting of authentic emotions and sense of belonging (Miller, 1997).

The sociocultural dyad consists of the following elements:

- Element 4: Self in sociocultural context. The experience of self as mirrored in larger social contexts in the family, extended family, community, and media.
- Element 5: Multiple layers of self. The experience of multiple layers of identity through awareness raising and feedback in caregiving relationships and through the salience of certain layers over others in the mirroring of important people in social contexts. Tatum (1997) offers a useful framework of seven layers of identity: ethnicity, gender, religion, sexual orientation, socioeconomic class, age, and ability.

Element One: Connection to Self

The infant starts out life experiencing many sensations/perceptions and feelings in his own skin. These may be perceptions and feelings of warmth and cold, hunger and satiety, sleep and alertness, sounds of the caregivers' voices and other environmental sounds, sight of the caregivers' faces when they are very close, textures of the skins that touch him, or textures of the materials in which he is held. He may feel collected when he is warmly held and gently rocked in response to his cries. He may experience himself quivering or startling in response to a sudden sound or touch. These are the early sensations and feelings, the early experiences of connecting with self in one's skin. It is not connection in any reflective sense, of course, but in terms of experiencing and being. The infant begins the journey of becoming aware and awake to himself through early sensory experiences in his body and early feelings about them. This is his early experience of presence or of being. Schafer (2004) has called such presence pure, unlabeled, unburdened awareness. Schafer also added another important, early, experiential component to this presence: joy, or the capacity to be open and drawn toward people and things in wonder without fear and without the impulse to reject.

Element Two: Dyadic Regulation of Self

The availability of a reliable, sensitive caregiver who reliably relieves distressing and overwhelming sensations and feelings lays the foundation for experiencing the regulation of sensations and feelings. It also lays the foundation for knowing who he is in a relationship context, of knowing that he is important and consistently cared for (or not), that his needs are met (or not), and whether or not he can trust his world. The human need for being seen and heard, cared for, respected, and honored begins in infancy and has been referred to as the need for mirroring that provides, in Alice Miller's (1997) words, the affective nourishment for the healthy growth of identity or sense of self. Miller speaks of early identity in terms of healthy self-feeling, which comes from authentic, natural contact with the feelings and needs within one's own skin. The experience of a self that is soothed, that can recover, and that is cared for can increasingly tolerate a wider range and intensity of these authentic feelings.

Element Three: Self in Relational Context

The experience of receiving reliable care, including dyadic regulation, becomes the basis of a positive sense of self in relational context. The lack of effective mirroring and affective nourishment leaves the self vulnerable to two pernicious forms of denial, grandiosity and depression, which can be fertile ground for emotional disturbance or illness. Miller (1997) presents and illustrates this idea with a fund of clinical information. Research in multicultural infant–family mental health repeatedly demonstrates that caregiver depression and other forms of mental illness can be significant risk factors for developing young children. When there is an absence of healthy self-feelings in the primary caregiver, the young child can be at risk for developing such self-feelings, but individual outcomes will vary on the basis of the balance of risk and protective factors in the family and context.

The accumulation of a positive balance of experience in the socioemotional triad (connection to self, dyadic regulation of self, and connection to self in relationship) yields a strong foundation of healthy self-feelings. This foundation includes enduring feelings of trust and balance in the rhythms of one's own body; relationships with others; feelings of security, safety, and bondedness; and feelings of belonging. This sense of belonging in early relationships is later generalized to family, work group, community, cultural group, nation, and species. Similarly, repeated experiences of (a) feeling overwhelmed by or disconnected from self through sensory processing difficulties or unmodulated intense feelings, (b) exposure to or experience of hidden or obvious traumas, and (c) lack of effective regulation of the resultant states by caregivers can result in various unfavorable outcomes for the emerging sense of self. These outcomes include the lack of reliable connection to authentic self-feelings and means of regulating them, lack of clarity about self in relationships, insecurity of attachments, excessive anxiety within one's skin and in relationships, and a sense of isolation in relationships and in social contexts.

Salvador Minuchin (Minuchin & Nichols, 1993) gave a fascinating account of the evolution of his early sociocultural identity. In early childhood, his influential older cousin made him believe that there was a special place in his brain where a bird resided and sang all the songs that he sang. Even in older years, he held onto this idea that a bird in his cerebellum was the originator of his poetry and songs, as well as the humor and metaphors that he used in his role as a clinician—those things that he identified as being at the core of his self. But the idea evolved. He realized that if he was this bird, the relationships in which he was embedded were the song, and that every time he sang the same song, it differed depending on the context in which he sang it. This idea illustrates, graphically, the idea that the self is dynamic and relational. Winnicott spoke of the self as a sacred, incommunicado element (Phillips, 1988), and so it may be, within our grasp and then just beyond it, connecting us to the power within us and to our interconnectedness with all that is around us.

Element Four: Self in Sociocultural Context

The components of ethnic/cultural knowledge, self-identification, constancy, role behaviors, and feelings or preferences develop gradually in the early childhood years and come to be experienced as a continuous and constant part of the self (Bernal, Knight, Ocampo, Garza, & Cota, 1993; Ocampo, Knight, & Bernal, 1997). Positive ownership of this identity is more complex for disadvantaged children, who may be poor, disabled, minorities, or of mixed heritage. Failure to own one's identity is reflected in internalized racism and other painful "isms" or forms of self-discrimination and disempowerment. The process of positive ownership of identity is related to positive self-image and sense of self-worth, and these are related to better social adjustment and school performance (Ogbu, 1989). Majority children also may experience the challenges of creating a healthy self-view in the realities of a dynamic, plural context. These challenges are intensified through aversive racism (Dovidio, Glick, & Rudman, 2005), the failure to reflectively examine racist beliefs and practices because of the belief that racism is so aversive to oneself that one cannot be involved with it. This belief can prevent an individual from unpacking the invisible knapsack of privilege (McIntosh, 1998) and can leave aspects of the self unprepared for open, egalitarian interaction with sociocultural diversity.

In the following passage, Beverly Tatum (1997) eloquently articulated what it means to include sociocultural diversity in the understanding of a young child's identity:

> *Who am I? The answer depends in large part on who the world around me says I am. Who do my parents say I am? Who do my peers say I am? What messages are reflected back to me in the faces and voices of my teachers, my neighbours, store clerks? What do I learn from the media about myself? How am I represented in the cultural images around me? Or am I missing altogether? As the social scientist Charles Cooley pointed out long ago, other people are the mirror in which we see ourselves.* (p. 18)

In toddlerhood, when language develops in leaps and bounds and the toddler gains the ability to communicate, absorb, and express more complex meanings, he may hear and take in who he is "just like" in the family or how his facial features, gait, or mannerisms remind others in the family of someone. With an overwhelming percentage of parents of toddlers in the full-time workforce, day care and preschool experience is common for a large proportion of our nation's toddlers. They may begin to hear about color, gender, ability, and other differences among them and their peers. In trips to the supermarket, the park, or even the doctor's office, they may hear about such things as well. In their research, Derman-Sparks, Higa, and Sparks (1980) found that young children are, first and foremost, interested in physical characteristics of themselves and others and, second, on readily observable cultural characteristics such as language and dress. Therefore, the query of a young child quoted by this research team makes sense. The child asked if he "had to be [B]lack" (Derman-Sparks et al., 1980, p. 6), considering that he wanted so much to be a chief of paramedics and his favorite TV program showed all the paramedics and firefighters as White. The same team's quote of yet another young child also makes sense. The child asked, "Why are there no [B]lack supermen?" Similarly, my middle child's comment in early childhood—"I wish I was [W]hite, then I would look better"—was painful, but it made sense (Banerjee, 2000). The fact that he made this statement within a few months of first entering school is significant. This story continues as follows:

It was ironic for my husband and I that this child of ours should have any misgivings about how he looked. Of all our handsome children, we have sometimes discussed how he is perhaps the most blessed with good looks . . . . we have in fact jested among ourselves that he has the makings of a dapper, dashing young man and worried about what troubles that could bring him and us someday!

So I introduced him to the idea of beauty lying in the eyes of the beholder . . . . we experimented with each of our notions about who looked good. . . . I said that in my mind color had nothing to do with looking good or not. He considered the idea enthusiastically. I told him that some people thought differently than I did.

We talked about this idea off and on for several days and went on to talking about being good. I told him that that also had nothing to do with color or with looking good.

Some weeks later, he was getting dressed and I was helping him freshen his face and comb his hair. When we were done and he was looking into the mirror, I asked, what do you think? How do you look? . . . . He immediately responded with I look good . . . and I don't have to worry about being [W]hite, huh? . . . . Then he said, Mama, I love the way you talk with me about these things."
—Banerjee, 2000 (pp. 16–17)

Admittedly, my son is socioemotionally attuned, precocious, and expressive, but conversations such as this that I have had with children of mixed heritage (Indian, Anglo, German, and Swedish American) have sensitized me to how much very young children can and do absorb about their sociocultural identities from the mirrors of their societies and community.

Exciting new research reported in *Science* is beginning to demonstrate the interplay between our genes and environment with regards to the way in which we deal with diversity and difference. In a study conducted by Olsson, Ebert, Banaji, and Phelps (2005), nervous arousal measured by sweat gland activity was higher for both African Americans and Caucasian Americans in response to the sight of a stranger of another race. This response was nearly absent among those of either race with histories of interracial dating. The interplay of possible genetic priming and natural human caution around the unfamiliar, along with unconsciously held biases against the different, are offered as explanations for these findings. We may, indeed, have been wired to stay in similar-looking groups and avoid different-looking groups for purposes of survival, explaining genetic priming for a natural human alertness around difference. However, we have shifted enormously in our evolutionary history as a species in our current global world. In this world difference, "not sameness" is becoming the norm (Suarez-Orozco & Qin-Hilliard, 2004). Herein lies our sociocultural and adaptation challenge. This research points to the possibility that active interaction across diversity can affect and change the nervous alertness and caution, perhaps through changed perceptions and attitudes. In my previous writing, I offered insights on the issue of not only dating but also exchange, dialogue, and interaction of a variety of types and referred to it as processes of *socioemotional integration* at collective, relational, and individual levels (Banerjee, 2002).

Working constructively with a historically fractured sociocultural identity is in our interest and in the interest of our young children. They have an endogenous curiosity about their social worlds, an inclination to interact with, make sense of, and categorize them as soon as their cognitive capacities allow them to do so (Banerjee, 2000). Histories of oppression and injustice are as old as humankind and may have some connection to the fearfulness and caution toward difference that we may have been primed for in evolution and that may have intensified through social experiences of oppression. Increasing our awareness and connections to the multiple layers of sociocultural identity that each of us has serves as a possible route for adaptively embracing the shift toward difference in a diverse global community.

Element Five: Multiple Layers of Self

Dialogue on multiple layers of identity is gaining momentum in the professional multicultural literature. Bringing the questions of early sociocultural identity into this discussion means that looking at the infant and young child's emerging sociocultural identity in sociocultural, sociohistorical, and sociopolitical contexts. It means that we actively and proactively deal with difference and complexity, the inevitable challenges awaiting those in our nurseries in our interconnected, global world.

My own ongoing reflections on these matters reveal to me the following motivations and organizing dimensions in the multiple layers of my identity:

> *In the process of immigration to the United States, I have personally lost the privilege of being among those who get to name everything. It is a privilege that I have chosen to lose. In my pre-immigration life, I had the experience of a social context in which privilege came for no good reason. In my post-immigration life, I have the experience of a social context where discrimination comes for no good reason. The place in which I now stand in the fullness of the experiences of my life, with access to*

both kinds of contexts, I own as a unique place from which to give voice to the cause of democratic social change.
—Banerjee, 2002 (pp. 14–15)

Indeed, privilege and discrimination are made possible because of one another. Both are products of a paradigm and a mindset defined by hierarchy and exclusion, in which value is accorded to a few at the expense of many. Privilege and discrimination are representations of an unintegrated paradigm in which totality of reality, the subjective and objective, are not included and in which partial connections result in ourselves and in our relationships with the diversity of relationships in the world. By some very sound scientific assessments, we, in following this path, are paving the way for our annihilation, with global warming serving as a clear signal of which even young children are being made aware through preschool projects.

Tatum (1997) refers to seven layers of identity: ethnicity, gender, religion, sexual orientation, socioeconomic class, age, and ability. In addition to bringing to our own awareness and comfort zones the language of our multiple layers of identity and introducing young children to the same, there are other important aspects to approaching sociocultural identity in this way. Examination of multiple layers and aspects in one's own identity leads to the inevitable facing of questions of one's own privileges and oppressions. The balance of the two may vary greatly by the circumstances, gender, color, and other differences between individuals. However the fundamental reality of both types of experience lies within the realm of experience of each of us. Therefore, engaging with it purposefully and constructively can increase our capacity for empathy with ourselves, with others, and with their struggles in society. It can increase our understanding of the complexity and depth of the effect of sociocultural factors in an individual's life experience. It can help us facilitate the development of an infant/young child's sociocultural identity with greater awareness. It can remove us from taking only a group-based view of diversity, thus forsaking the complexity of individual experiences or vice versa, and it can allow us to take both levels of reality into account. This way, we are in a better position to take an informed view of group history and perspective and to balance it with the ways in which an individual's situation aligns with or departs from it. For example, a majority person may examine, own, and voice the unjust privileges that have come their way from being a member of their group in society as well as the oppressions that they have experienced in different aspects of their personal lives because of familial, relational, and personal factors. A minority person can examine, own, and voice the oppressions that have visited them and that continue to do so on a daily basis because of their group membership as well as the privileges that they have experienced in their personal life, relationships, and family. A more holistic perspective keeps us from generating new prejudices and polarizations in the struggle for social justice and opens us to humane consideration and connection with one another's experiences. The more constructive and hopeful an adult's experience with these challenging issues, the greater the likelihood that they can actively integrate it and consciously pass it on in the socializing of their children.

Encouraging young children to identify with different aspects of their identities is a way of helping them value diversity and heterogeneity, not because it has any absolute value but because it represents healthy self-owning in current-day, heterogenous societies and has adaptive value (Banerjee, 2000). It also teaches flexibility, a psychological quality that builds resilience and well-being. This flexibility allows young children to experience the fact that borders can be permeable, "going beyond respecting differences to meaningful sharing, partaking and two-way absorbing of cultural diversity" (Banerjee, 2000, p. 18). This kind of exchange is illustrated in Kindler's (1994) story of her young son Jan's experience growing up in Canada. He was so absorbed by a chance exposure to the Haida art of the First Nations of the Northwest that when his teacher requested that the class engage in multicultural sharing, Jan shared this rather than something from his Polish-American heritage. His mother saw his deep and genuine involvement with the bold depictions of ravens, killer whales, frogs, and eagles in this Native American form of art. She eloquently articulated her understanding by saying that his forming identity at that time and thence forth has continued to include "fragments of Northwest Coast First Nations heritage to the extent that he . . . understood and constructed his version of it" (Kindler, 1994, p. 59). Perhaps in such seeds of socioemotional integration of diverse peoples lies the hope of adaptation to our present and future challenge in a global world in which diversity—not sameness—is the norm.

As Tatum (1997) points out, reflecting on one's own experiences of becoming aware of differences is a helpful starting point. I remember an experience in early preschool having to do with *physiognomy*, or what we may more commonly call race. It would be helpful to have had memories from infancy, but my neurophysiology does not cooperate. Research categorizes infant memories as implicit (Siegal, 1999) and not readily accessible for recall. To put some sociocultural context around my memories, I grew up as an Indian in India, relatively privileged, in a Brahmin, upper-middle-class family from Bengal. Indian society has long had more diversity in it than all of Europe combined, and this diversity has been kept alive through the use of numerous native languages, cultural rituals, and socialization practices. On one occasion when I was in my early preschool years, I noticed a couple in Kolkata whose physical appearance looked, to me, to be quite different from one another. I curiously asked my mother how they could be a couple when they did not look like one another. Her spontaneous response was that it was not necessary to look like one another in order to be a couple; this response was an early gift of ease with diversity from which I believe I have drawn in my later experiences with immigration and marriage to a White, Anglo-Saxon American. Tatum, an African American woman, reports a very similar incident in her parenting of one of her young sons in which her response was "they don't have to match" (p. 33). The striking similarity of our experiences across cultures and cohorts—in fact, halfway across the world—says something about certain common dilemmas in the form of common questions that can be faced by parents and children in dealing with diversity in the early years.

Young children not only want to be seen and heard for who they are but they also notice the myriad differences in them and around them from toddlerhood. They seek explanations for their observations (Tatum, 1997), and they need their questions to be heard and responded to. Awareness and engagement with these questions and experience and support in exploring them are necessary components in adults feeling that they can engage with them with their children. Self-reflection or guided self-reflections in groups can reveal many interesting themes in people's experiences. Tatum (1997) identifies some of the themes in peoples' early experiences with diversity, including curiosity, fear, avoidance, mixed messages, terror, sadness, active bigotry, and so forth. She notes the absence of themes of joy, excitement, delight, and so forth, and perhaps this is why we are so often scared into a code of silence in these uncomfortable conversations about diversity. Yet, it is important to realize that the opportunity for an active transition from societies organized around sameness to societies organized around variety and difference is here. It is an evolutionary, species-level opportunity.

Tone of conversations about diversity is perhaps even more important than the content itself, for it contains powerful information about feelings. Congruence between the verbal and nonverbal layers of message is very important in communicating effectively with young children about these issues. Tatum's (1997) model of facing difficult questions such as the history of slavery with her own children is an excellent one. She emphasized the importance of not worrying her child that (a) he would be vulnerable to such a fate; (b) their African American ancestors were victims but not passive victims—they resisted actively; and (c) not all White people were unjust—there were White abolitionists, too. This is an excellent model for several reasons. It faces, rather than avoids, difficult questions; it answers them honestly and thoughtfully, with care for the young child's sensibilities and capacities; and it presents the picture with complexity and realism, not dogma or stereotype.

Lest it be implied that diversity is a minority concern for the socialization of minority children, it is important to note that the definition of *majority* and *minority* is dynamic and, in parts of this society and in parts of the globe, will be shifting more quickly in the coming decades than in decades past. Diversity is part of each of our futures and is each of our concern. The challenges associated with facing privilege—such as unpacking the invisible knapsack of White privilege (McIntosh, 1998), of the relative privilege of lighter skin color, and other arbitraries—is equally vital to the preparation and empowerment of all young children for healthy interaction in a diverse world. Sensitizing young children to these aspects of themselves and caring about social justice works, even in early childhood with adult guidance (Derman-Sparks & the ABC Task Force, 1989; Derman-Sparks et al., 1980).

All young children can be helped not only through adult dialogue and interaction but also through genuinely caring, respectful relationships with people quite similar and rather different to themselves and their families. Young children can discover and become familiar with diversity through its meaningful representation in art and music in their surroundings and through activities, stories, mythologies, and celebrations shared in their environments. Rhythm and pace of speaking, of thinking, of daily living, and of music (White, personal communication, June 10, 2005) can differ across microcultures and macrocultures and are very important to experience and understand to prevent premature labeling or mislabeling. Finally, the journey toward embracing our inherent diversities and passing them on to young children is, like all central journeys, an ongoing and abiding one. The deeper that adults' pursue passion for and engagement in issues of social justice and equity, the more active and plentiful will be the opportunities and modeling for young children to do the same.

The Five Elements of Sociocultural Identity and Development

The elements in the socioemotional triad enter the infant's experience at birth and are connected to the experience of establishing a balance of felt trust over distrust (Erikson, 1963) of the self within the skin and in caregiving relationships. The elements in the sociocultural dyad enter the child's experience as he moves from infancy to toddlerhood, begins to experience himself as a member of his first society (family and beyond), and explores experiences of autonomy versus doubt and shame and initiative versus guilt (Erikson, 1963).

Experience of his first society or family and his larger society or community is hardly possible in our diverse society and global community without the experience of diversity, with its complexity and complex history. If we are moved to consider such a perspective as too heavy and burdensome in the innocent early years of infancy and early childhood, we are succumbing to the denial of painful reality, denial that cuts us off from our inherent capacities for experiencing this perspective and making healthy connections with it. Therefore, the question of early sociocultural identity is approached within the history and context of that identity in society.

Questions for Accessing the Sociocultural Identity of the Infant and Young Child
Present Moment, Child-Focused Questions

1. *If you were to describe what you have learned about who your infant is from all your experiences of caring for him and playing with him, enjoying him, what would you say?*

2. *If you were to describe what you have learned about who your infant is from your experiences of observing him and observing him with others, what would you say?*

3. *As you watch over your toddler, follow him, keep him safe, and watch the world opening up for him as he explores it, who would you say he is and who is he becoming?*

4. When he communicates what he enjoys, what distresses him, what he needs, who does he tell you that he is?

5. What messages is your child getting about who he is from your family and from other important parts of his social environment (extended family, preschool/day care, media)? How is he responding to these messages?

6. If you were to describe the different layers of your child's identity (color, gender, abilities, preferences, socioeconomic class, religion, geographical region, ethnicity), how would you describe him? What messages do you give him about these different layers? What messages do you want to give him?

7. Which of these layers are currently most important to you in facilitating his development? What messages do you want to give him about these layers, and how?

Historical, Caregiver-Focused Questions

1. If you look back to your early childhood, how far back do your memories take you? If you go to the earliest remembered times, what is your memory of who you were, of your early, emerging sense of self?

2. In what ways is your child like you were and are, and in what ways is he different?

3. Who does your child remind you of? In what ways is he like this person, and in what ways is he different?

4. What are your earliest memories of yourself in which you were aware of your race, color, religion, class, or other aspects of sociocultural identity?

5. What are your feelings about these early memories? How were these feelings handled? Did anyone help you with them? How did that go?

6. What resources did you have in dealing with issues of identity and the complexities and confusions of difference in the early years of your childhood? What do you wish you had?

7. What resources on dealing with the complexities of difference in the early years do you want to give your child? What are some of the ways in which you want to pass on these resources, messages, and lessons?

8. *What are the different layers of your identity that are important to you? What are your resources (positive experiences, family support, group support) and barriers (experiences of distrust, shame, or hostility; immigration and loss of context; lack of family support; lack of salience/visibility or awareness in the community, media) in passing these layers on to your young child?*

Circle Two: Primary Caregiving Relationships

If attachment research had its origins in non-western cultures, we suspect that qualities like proper demeanour and sunao would be considered universal consequences of security.
—Rothbaum & Morelli, 2005 (p. 107)

Human infancy has a relatively long period of dependency on primary caregiving relationships. Maturational processes unfold in the context of these relationships, and the quality of these relationships set the foundation for the quality of the young child's relationships with others. The field of multicultural infant–family mental health was founded on the premise of seeing the infant and young child's well-being in this relational context (Fraiberg, Adelson, & Shapiro, 1975). An enormous amount of research, which was conducted on the basis of the same premise, has occurred in the area of attachment and has linked attachment very strongly to later well-being.

Bowlby's (1953, 1969, 1973, 1980) insights on attachment that is placed in an ethological context and Ainsworth, Blehar, Waters, and Wall's (1978) continuation of that work in a cross-cultural context set off a fire in the bellies of scholars, researchers, and practitioners in the western world who were concerned with early development. The list of contributors to the meticulous body of work that has developed in this area requires no introduction. However, diversity has not yet received serious attention in this work. The principle of unity of developmental processes seems to have been a driving thrust instead. Culture, from this perspective, becomes nonfundamental. The variations it causes are seen to represent differences in appearance only; therefore, constructs and tools are taken from one culture and are applied in others. These other cultures include those who are perceived as less developed, with fewer material resources and less familiar cultures. As a result, meaning—the unique and treasured capacity of our species (Cole, 2005)—and the variations of meaning that affect motives, behavior patterns, objectives, and outcomes of attachment in our diverse world are barely accounted for and seem little understood in this dense knowledge base. Attunement to culturally specific processes in attachment and the political effects of missing these nuances for those in socially oppressed groups is surprisingly undeveloped.

Subjectivity is an inevitable part of every endeavor, and denied subjectivity leads not only to partial illumination of reality but also to unawareness of what is being missed in the data and how one's subjective biases are shaping the constructs and measures that researchers are using to collect the data. These realities are important to consider because they have to do with an influential knowledge base about dynamics at the beginning of human life and at the core of human survival and well-being. As James Baldwin has been quoted as saying (Tatum, 1997), we might be able to change that which we face up to, but we have no chance to change that which we do not face up to. Here again a fundamental epistemological question becomes important to ask. What are the costs of overvaluing objective methods of inquiry and distrusting the depths and discipline of subjective processes of inquiry and the inevitable interactions between the two? Can the subjective inputs be looked at in any way other than as noise/distraction/impurity in our quest to grasp the nature of phenomena?

There is new hope in the steady trickle in the knowledge base caused by the work of Rothbaum and colleagues (Rothbaum & Kakinuma, 2004; Rothbaum & Morelli, 2005; Rothbaum, Rosen, Ujiie, & Uchida, 2002; Rothbaum, Weisz, Pott, Miyake, & Morelli, 2000). These researchers have begun to demonstrate the kinds of questions that we need to ask to get beneath premature notions of universality of attachment theory components and open up, instead, to the complexity and variability of its components. They have put culture and the value systems deriving from it at the center—not the periphery—of their inquiry, and, by synthesizing their own empirical data and the findings of others across cultures, they have offered many interesting insights. Because value systems influence socialization processes and parenting behaviors, the objectives or socialization goals of attachment vary with culture. In cultures where the socialization process in the nursery is geared toward interdependence, emotional closeness and dependence in the infant and young child may be rewarded. This reward may manifest in prolonged skinship (Rothbaum et al., 2005), cosleeping, and, later, weaning (Carlson & Harwood, 2000) and sensitivity to the child's cues and needs through sophisticated reading of nonverbal cues and proactive, anticipatory engagement in fulfilling them. This gives the infant the early experience of being intimately known within her skin by empathic caregivers and family members. She experiences that her caregivers' commitment to her is unbounded and unconditional (Rothbaum & Kakinuma, 2004). The culturally sanctioned and directed purpose of this experience is not only to be prepared to have similar proactive, anticipatory engagement with the nonverbally communicated needs of close others but also to deepen capacities for empathic understandings of them and strengthen tendencies to create and seek harmony in relationships. Through such socialization, awareness of the nuances and nonverbal climate of the relational context develops naturally. The objective of such a culturally influenced attachment process is also to adhere to circular life-cycle expectations. These expectations are that parents invest in personal care for their young children and elderly parents simultaneously and closely and that the young child grows up to do the same. It makes intuitive sense that in such a context, longer and more indulgent (Nwoye, 2006) periods of dependence may be very helpful to prepare for these developmental goals and create the type of bonds that will ensure them.

In cultural contexts in which nutrition, health, and safety concerns of parents are relatively higher, more physical control is found to be normative, or more caregiving attention in response to negative, not positive, actions may be normative (Carlson & Harwood, 2003; Rothbaum & Morelli, 2005). What can be experienced and seen as intrusive and insecurity-producing in one cultural context is experienced very differently in another because of the protective meaning attributed to it. In cultures and families in which the socialization process in the nursery is geared toward the socialization goal of independence, parental behavior will be rewarding of young children practicing autonomy and independent action, exploring the environment within safe limits, and acting upon that environment. Thus a child who picks up a ball and throws it may be recognized with enthusiasm and warm tones by her mother and father. She gets to experience what it means to do something in her culture. She gets to feel that she is doing it. Her mother's actions are in response to her actions, not in anticipation of them and so, for her, being nonverbally read and empathically known within her skin by a caregiver is not the experience of availability, sensitivity, and responsivity. Taking some action in the world for herself or acting autonomously and being recognized for it is. As her forays into her world grow, she needs to rest in the trust of her caregivers. This trust in reliable connections with significant others frees her to explore and seek new opportunities (Rothbaum & Kakinuma, 2004).

The ease and fluency with interconnectedness of the child preparing to manage and carry a complex, close network of relationships through life is very different in quality from the lightness of the trust of the child preparing to make her own way in the world with a nucleus of trust in herself and in those whom her life touches. This child who is encouraged to act upon the world will more than likely be regulated by her mother by more distal forms of contact, such as eye contact, more often and at an earlier age. She herself will respond in more distal ways, such as with social referencing. This child is also likely to be socialized with linear life-cycle expectations, wherein her parents are invested in the close, personal care of their children until they reach maturity, after which the children are expected to be autonomous and, in time, take care of their own children in a similar way. Once again, it makes intuitive sense that when independence is desired, it is rewarded and provided early so that it helps the young person focus on her agency in the world. At the same time, individual family members in this cultural context may experience and adhere to more interdependent socialization values, and the same can be said of individual families in interdependent cultural contexts. Broad generalizations have to be qualified by the reality of individual cases.

Besides the matter of a cultural focus on interdependence or independence in child rearing as this focus affects attachment processes, the nature of autonomy itself can vary culturally. The vision of an active, curious, confident, outgoing young child may be what autonomy looks like and is recognized to be in one cultural context, and a calm, open, receptive, interactive child may be what autonomy looks like in the other culture. The latter perspective can come from a context in which an assertive person is seen as "immature and uncultivated" (Fiske et al., 1998, p. 923, as cited in Rothbaum &

Morelli, 2005). Attachment outcomes of competence in such contexts can be understood to mean concerning oneself with furthering the goals of close others as well as oneself, contributing to society through turning to the wisdom and experience of elders, acknowledging the shoulders on which an individual stands, acceptance and fulfillment of social roles (Rothbaum & Morelli, 2005), and coordinating the needs of others as well as oneself (Kitayama & Markus, 1994; Roland, 1988). In taking into account the complexities of culture, sociopolitical and sociohistorical factors such as histories of brutality, oppression, and losses from natural and human-created factors, as well as the presence of varied and unique sociocultural resource factors such as alternative caregivers (Rothbaum & Morelli, 2005) and extended family networks, are important to keep in mind.

The shift in domestic culture from homogenization to greater openness to diversity means that each young child and each young caregiving dyad has more opportunities to discover the myriad cultural influences that are a part of them. The ease and pervasiveness of technology-facilitated access to the globe breaks the isolation of a continent and its people separated from others by geography and policies. This provides access for many young children, dyads, and families to new influences, familiar and unfamiliar. These are the opportunities for connection that hold promise for the globe becoming a smaller place, where the richness of diversity can be integrated through collaborative means rather than denied and truncated through fear-generating, hierarchy/power/greed-driven, oppressive means.

Returning to the caregiving dyad, connections between the temperaments of the young child and caregiver that fit or do not fit (Chess & Thomas, 1996) are useful to consider. *Fit* emphasizes the notion of relationship and reciprocity and the ways in which it can be strengthened and maintained. The quality of the caregiving relationship has been given its due place in the *DC:0–3R* (ZERO TO THREE, 2005) on Axis II. This axis follows the first axis in which the criteria of clinical disorders are spelled out, and this axis exemplifies the multicultural infant–family mental health approach to young children functioning in caregiving context. This shift from the structure of Axis II in the *DSM-IV-TR* (American Psychiatric Association, 2000) on individually defined, long-standing personality disorders to relationship disorders represents a shift toward understanding mental disorder etiology and course in complex, relationship contexts. Venturing further into this complexity can result in adding variations in family cultures and broader cultures of identification. Resources in the form of training materials and trainings, colleagues who are well-versed in the challenges of integrating diversity considerations in their work who have depth of understanding in particular cultures, and commitment to multicultural competence are essential companions in journeying toward this complexity.

Circle Three: Caregivers

The caregivers in the nursery carry the ordinary and daunting responsibility for the development and well-being of young children. These children are their future and ours. Two caregiver factors have been identified as being of particular relevance to the care of infants and young children. These factors relate to caregiver well-being and availability and are caregivers' mental health and caregivers' early caregiving or attachment history. Caregiver history of mental illness and its effect on the caregiver's relationship with the child and family members constitutes an important part of the infant and young child's genetic and environmental history. The caregiving relationship provides the caregiver with both the opportunity and the challenge of becoming a mother (Stern & Bruschweiler-Stern, 1998) or a parent, as well as reacquainted with early experiences of attachment and fit. However, awareness and reflection on this history can offer the caregiver the choice to thoughtfully use similar and different strategies with their young child.

Growth is invariably an intertwined, bidirectional, depth-giving process. We encounter opportunities for growth in parenting a newborn, in working as a professional who facilitates secure attachment in newborns and caregivers, in creating programs serving such dyads and families, in researching nuances of relationship processes, and creating policies affecting social priorities related to these processes. Research on caregiver well-being and attachment history indicates the strong tendency for human caregivers to go where they have gone before or, in other words, to repeat the past. We take our time as a species, it seems, to learn from the lessons of history. However, given the support, knowledge, and connections necessary for reflection on difficult and painful experiences, we also show the capacity and the courage to face them, the flexibility to heal and to forge new relationship patterns with new generations in our care (Siegal & Hartzell, 2003).

Ultimately, we can take others to the new places we go to ourselves, or we can inspire them by our own efforts to grow. Experience opens the doorway to growth and its transformative power. Professional experience teaches that, although trained eyes and ears can spot the signatures of early history in old defenses, working effectively with caregivers toward change requires strong relationships. These are relationships of well-established trust, respect, boundaries, and fine-tuned assessments of timing based on sound knowledge that make deeper journeys possible. Not every parent will be willing or ready to work on their own history, and not every clinician will inspire them to. Not every program will focus on underlying factors such as parental history, nor will every policy initiative get behind providing access to parental mental health services. Not every research study will consider the caregiver's past or how that past manifests itself in the present.

Regardless of training, if professionals know the terrain themselves, they can encourage caregivers to take reparative journeys and peers to create institutional infrastructures, cultures, and climates to support these journeys. Bowen's (1985) call to professionals to make the journey back home, and the reflective supervision underpinnings of connection, reflection, and regularity (Fenichel, 1992), speak of entry into such terrain. The experience of holding dialectical tensions in the range of human emotions, the shades of bright and dark emotions, can offer another route through increasing affect tolerance. The experience of hearing and telling stories or narratives in which subjective and objective information are richly integrated can offer another route through access to personal–cultural meaning. The simultaneous experience of intrapersonal/interpersonal connection and detachment can offer yet another route through the deepening of breath and stillness.

References

Ainsworth, M. D. S., Blehar, M. C., Waters, E., & Wall, S. (1978). *Patterns of attachment: A psychological study of the strange situation.* Hillsdale, NJ: Erlbaum.

American Psychiatric Association. (2000). *Diagnostic and statistical manual of mental disorders–IV TR* (4th ed.). Washington, DC: Author.

Banerjee, L. (1989, December). *Mother Infant Support Team (MIST): A program for preventing child abuse and neglect in severe high risk infants.* Paper presented at the Sixth Biennial National Training Institute of the National Center for Clinical Infant Programs, Washington, DC.

Banerjee, L. (1990, October). *Effective programs for the prevention of child abuse and neglect 0–5: Healthy Start and mother infant support team.* Paper presented at the meeting of the Family Resource Coalition, Chicago.

Banerjee, L. (2000). Through a child's eyes: What's in a name and other thoughts on social categorization in America. *The Community Psychologist, 33*(2), 16–18.

Banerjee, L. (2002). Psychology and the reach of multiculturalism in American culture. In E. Davis-Russell (Ed.), *Handbook of multicultural education, research, intervention, and training* (pp. 3–19). San Francisco: Jossey-Bass.

Bernal, M. E., Knight, G. P., Garza, C. A., Ocampo, K. A., & Cota, M. K. (1993). Development of Mexican American Identity. In M. E. Bernal & G. P. Knight (Eds.), *Ethnic identity formation and transmission among Hispanics and other minorities* (pp. 31–46). Albany, NY: State University of New York Press.

Bowen, M. (1985). *Family therapy in clinical practice.* Northvale, NJ: Jason Aronson.

Bowlby, J. (1953). *Child care and the growth of love.* London: Penguin Books.

Bowlby, J. (1969). *Attachment* [Attachment and Loss Series, Vol. 1]. New York: Basic Books.

Bowlby, J. (1973). *Separation: Anxiety and anger* [Attachment and Loss Series, Vol. 2]. New York: Basic Books.

Bowlby, J. (1980). *Loss: Sadness and depression* [Attachment and Loss Series, Vol. 3]. New York: Basic Books.

Carlson, V. J., & Harwood, R. L. (2000). Understanding and negotiating cultural differences concerning early developmental competence. *Zero to Three, 20*, 19–24.

Carlson, V. J., & Harwood, R. L. (2003). Attachment, culture, and the caregiving system: The cultural patterning of everyday experiences among Anglo and Puerto Rican mother–infant pairs. *Infant Mental Health Journal, 24*, 53–73.

Chess, S., & Thomas, A. (1996). *Temperament: Theory and practice.* Philadelphia: Brunner/Mazel.

Clinton, H. R. (1996). *It takes a village and other lessons children teach us.* New York: Simon & Schuster.

Cole, M. (2005). *Developmental science: An advanced textbook.* Mahwah, NJ: Erlbaum.

Csikszentmihalyi, M. (1990). *Flow: The psychology of optimal experience.* New York: Harper Perennial.

Day, M., & Parlakian, R. (2003). *How culture shapes social–emotional development: Implications for practice in infant–family programs.* Washington, DC: ZERO TO THREE.

Derman-Sparks, L., & the ABC Task Force. (1989). *Anti-bias curriculum tools for empowering young children.* Washington, DC: National Association for the Education of Young Children.

Derman-Sparks, L., Higa, C. T., & Sparks, B. (1980). Children, race, and racism: How race awareness develops. *Interracial Books for Children, 11*, 3–9.

Dovidio, J. F., Glick, P. G., & Rudman, L. (Eds.). (2005). *On the nature of prejudice: Fifty years after Allport.* Malden, MA: Blackwell.

Erikson, E. (1963). *Childhood and society.* New York: W. W. Norton.

Fenichel, E. (Ed.). (1992). *Learning through supervision and mentorship how to support the development of infants, toddlers and their families: A source book.* Washington, DC: ZERO TO THREE.

Fraiberg, S., Adelson, E., & Shapiro, V. (1975). Ghosts in the nursery. *Journal of the American Academy of Child Psychiatry, 14*, 387–421.

Goleman, Daniel. (1995). *Emotional intelligence.* New York: Bantam Books.

Greenspan, S. I., & Benderly, B. L. (1997). *The growth of the mind and the endangered origins of intelligence.* Reading, MA: Addison-Wesley.

Greenspan, S. I., DeGangi, G. A., & Wieder, S. (2001). *The Functional Emotional Assessment Scale (FEAS) for infancy and early childhood: Clinical and research applications.* Bethesda, MD: Interdisciplinary Council on Developmental and Learning Disorders.

Greenspan, S. I., & Wieder, S. (1998). *The child with special needs: Encouraging intellectual and emotional growth.* Reading, MA: Perseus Books.

Guerin, P. J., Fogarty, T. F., Fay, L. F., & Kautto, J. G. (1996). *Working with relationship triangles: The one-two-three of psychotherapy.* New York: Guilford Press.

Heffron, M. C. (2005). Reflective supervision in infant, toddler, and preschool work. In K. M. Finello (Ed.), *The handbook of training and practice in infant and preschool mental health* (pp. 114–136). San Francisco: Jossey-Bass.

Kindler, A. M. (1994, July). Children and the culture of a multicultural society. *Art Education, 47*(4), 54–60.

Kitayama, S., & Markus, H. R. (1994). Culture and self: How culture influences the way we view ourselves. In D. Matsumoto (Ed.), *People: Psychology from a cultural perspective* (pp. 17–37). Prospect Heights, IL: Waveland Press.

McIntosh, P. (1998). White privilege: Unpacking the invisible knapsack. In M. McGoldrick (Ed.), *Re-visioning family therapy, race, culture, and gender in clinical practice* (pp. 153–175). New York: Guilford Press.

Mead, M. (1935). *Sex and temperament in three primitive societies.* New York: William Morrow.

Miller, A. (1997). *The drama of the gifted child: The search for the true self.* New York: Basic Books.

Minuchin, S., & Nichols, M. (1993). *Family healing: Strategies for hope and understanding.* New York: Simon & Schuster.

Nwoye, A. (2006). A narrative approach to child and family therapy in Africa. *Contemporary Family Therapy, 28*(1), 1–23.

Ocampo, K. A., Knight, G. P., & Bernal, M. E. (1997). The development of cognitive abilities and social identities in children: The case of ethnic identity. *International Journal of Behavioral Development, 21,* 479–500.

Ogbu, J. (1989). *Cultural models and educational strategies of nondominant peoples* [1989 Catherine Molony Memorial Lecture]. New York: City College of New York Workshop Center.

Olsson, A., Ebert, J. P., Banaji, M. H., & Phelps, E. A. (2005, July 29). The role of social groups in the persistence of learned fear. *Science, 309,* 785–787.

Perry, B. (2003, May). *Nature and nurture of brain development.* Paper presented at the From Neurons to Neighborhoods Conference, Los Angeles, CA. Retrieved on December 18, 2006, from www.childtrauma.org

Phillips, A. (1988). *Winnicott.* London: Fontana Press.

Roland, A. (1988). *In search of self in India and Japan: Toward a cross-cultural psychology.* Princeton, NJ: Princeton University Press.

Rothbaum, F., & Kakinuma, M. (2004). Amae and attachment: Security in cultural context. *Human Development, 47,* 34–39.

Rothbaum, F., & Morelli, G. (2005). Attachment and culture: Reciprocal contributions of cross-cultural research and developmental psychology. In W. Friedlmeier, P. Chakkarath, & B. Schwarz (Eds.), *Culture and human development: The importance of cross-cultural research for the social sciences* (pp. 99–123). New York: Psychology Press.

Rothbaum, F., Rosen, K., Ujiie, T., & Uchida, N. (2002). Family systems theory, attachment theory, and culture. *Family Process, 41,* 328–350.

Rothbaum, F., Weisz, S., Pott, M., Miyake, K., & Morelli, G. (2000). Attachment and culture: Security in the United States and Japan. *American Psychologist, 55,* 1093–1104.

Schafer, W. (2004). The infant as reflection of soul: The time before there was a self. *Zero to Three, 24,* 4–8.

Shahmoon-Shanok, R. S., Gilkerson, L., Eggbeer, L., & Fenichel, E. (1995). *Reflective supervision: A relationship for learning* [Videotape and discussion guide]. Washington, DC: ZERO TO THREE.

Shahmoon-Shanok, R., Lapidus, C, Grant, M., Halpern, E., & Lamb-Parker, F. (2005). Apprenticeship, transformational enterprise, and the ripple effect. In K. M. Finello (Ed.), *The handbook of training and practice in infant and preschool mental health* (pp. 114–136). San Francisco: Jossey-Bass.

Siegal, D. J. (1999). *The developing mind.* New York: Guilford Press.

Siegal, D. J., & Hartzell, M. (2003). *Parenting from the inside out: How a deeper self-understanding can help you raise children who thrive.* New York: Penguin Putnam.

Sroufe, L. A., Egeland, B., Carlson, E. A., & Collins, W. A. (2005). *The development of the person.* New York: Guilford Press.

Stern, D. N., & Bruschweiler-Stern, N. (1998). *The birth of a mother: How the motherhood experience changes your life.* New York: Basic Books.

Suarez-Orozco, M. M., & Qin-Hilliard, D. B. (Eds.). (2004). *Globalization, culture, and education in the new millennium.* Berkeley and Los Angeles, CA: University of California Press.

Tatum, B. D. (1997). *"Why are all the Black kids sitting together in the cafeteria?" and other conversations about race.* New York: Basic Books.

ZERO TO THREE. (2005). *Diagnostic classification of mental health and developmental disorders of infancy and early childhood: Revised edition (DC:0–3R).* Washington, DC: Author.

CHAPTER 2
Family Systems and Culture

Leena Banerjee Brown

Circle Four: Family Systems and Culture, An Introduction

Family systems therapy revolutionized psychotherapy by its focus on the present-day interpersonal context, thus locating psychological health and dysfunction in the interpersonal space of relationships. Relevant traces of interior spaces and interpersonal history were to be found in this interpersonal space. Therefore, working experientially in the present context of emotionally influential relationships was a way of facilitating change in relationships and individuals and affecting their future development. This approach offered a new complexity, reduced blame on an individual for dysfunction, and began to take familial and sociocultural context into account in an integral way. In his classic style, Salvador Minuchin (S. Minuchin & Nichols, 1993), a founding parent of family therapy, reported on his early work using this approach. He visited a young, aggressive, out-of-control boy in the hospital (at a time when hospitalization was less cost forbidding and more liberally prescribed), and his mother immediately complained that she could not control him. Minuchin's question to her was simple and direct, then, why was she not in the hospital? In the end, after his interview with the mother and her son, he restated this perspective in a gentler way by saying that as long as she and her son did not fit, the boy would need the structure and holding of a hospital.

Relationships became the basic unit of definition. Gregory Bateson (1972), a pioneering thinker who propelled the field of family therapy forward, is quoted as raising his hand up at a seminar he was giving and asking how many fingers there were. The answer was five, but he said it was incorrect. A puzzled audience ventured a few other numbers as guesses before giving up. Bateson offered that the answer was that the question itself did not make sense because in the real world, there are only relationships between fingers—there are no fingers themselves. His message was to shift from objects to relationships (Capra, 1988). Current research in interpersonal neurobiology expands on the significance of this idea by offering that relationships affect brain development through the regulation of body states and emotions, the organization of memory, the capacity for interpersonal communication, and the creation of meaning (Siegal, 1999). Our internal and interpersonal spaces are integrally interconnected, an idea reasserted in family systems work but one as old as ancient philosophical treatises such as the Vedas and Upanishads (Aurobindo, 1972)—and perhaps older than that in human experience.

Interconnected, bidirectionally influential relationships make up a system of family relationships. There are identifiable patterns of interactions in this system as well as roles that are determined by it, by the individuals in it, and by larger cultural influences. *Bidirectional* or *reciprocal influences* means that if the mother in the family is recognized as the family spokesperson, the father is also recognized as the parent who gives his voice away to the mother. The different parts of a system are seen as theoretically equivalent (*equipotential*) in terms of their ability to effect change in the system. As agents of change, this ability underscores the importance of connecting meaningfully with all parts of the system or family, establishing respectful relationships with each person, and knowing each significant relationship. The idea that one can arrive at the same end place of change through different pathways is theoretically held to be true. Practically speaking, some pathways are better choices as starting points for catalyzing change. Take the case of a single-parent Hispanic American family in which the mother has two jobs. She is a support staff member in a long-term-care facility and also works in her child's school library. She has two children 10 years apart in age, a boy of 12 years and a girl of 2 years. She expects her son to help with numerous household and caregiving chores such as watching over his sister, taking her to the park, and so forth, because she says "he has to," meaning there is no one else to help. The 12-year-old is beginning to get really pushy and aggressive in his manner and tone with his sister, but he is protective of her with others and is supportive of his mother. To realign the parental role within the realistic resource limits of the family and to facilitate more optimal functioning, the clinician can take at least two courses of action in family therapy. The therapist can help the mother forge connections with extended family, neighbors, or community resources for respite care and parental support. At the same time, the therapist can support her in her challenging parenting role and help her see and differentiate the different developmental needs of each of her two children. Through such support, sensitization, and guidance, she can learn to free the 12-year-old to be his age but to also support her with specific, reasonable, delegated household and caregiving chores (as illustrated in the family maps in Figure 2.1).

Figure 2.1 Family maps for assessment and goal setting in two stages.

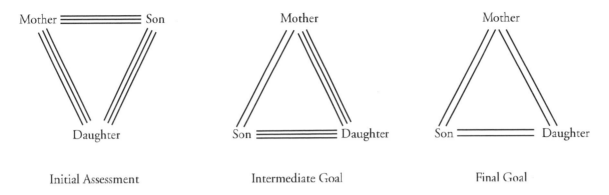

Initial Assessment   Intermediate Goal   Final Goal

This is support that their particular single-parent family structure cannot do without. In their reconfigured relationship, the mother can learn to model for her son appropriate ways to interact with his sister and to set limits with him when he overreaches in his attitude or behavior. Delegation implies that the authority rests on the mother's shoulders and that she assumes it. It implies that she is in charge, that she delegates specific tasks to her older child, that she supports him in implementing them, and that she sets limits on his behavior when necessary. If, on the other hand, the intervention process begins with a focus on the sibling relationship problems without first focusing on the authority structure problems between mother and son, the therapist may find it more difficult to address this issue later. From the mother and son's perspective, the change process may have initially validated the inappropriate hierarchy by not commenting on it, and, as painful as such dysfunctional family roles can be, the son may be loathe to give up his privileged position and the mother her helpless one.

Families are self-organizing and self-correcting. Like any system, they prefer homeostasis and go through inevitable transitions for developmental, life-cycle reasons such as the birth of a child or unpredictable, random occurrences such as an overseas job or relocation because of a natural disaster or war or loss of a family member. In these events, families weather transitions and reestablish a new homeostasis. Disruptions in homeostasis occur in shorter bursts compared with the more enduring states of homeostasis, whether this homeostasis is healthy and functional or unhealthy and dysfunctional.

Family therapy pays attention to the content as well as the process of family interactions. The interest is in the whole set of family communications, the said and the unsaid, the words and their meaning, the action and its context. Family therapy reaches for the metaphors that lie beneath family interactions or beneath any set of interactions. Bateson (1972) emphasized that metaphors are meta patterns and, therefore, are important tools for gaining knowledge about living things, as the living world is held together by interconnections. He asserted that metaphors, stories, narratives, and parables can contain the complexity of information that can tell about the experience of being alive. Metaphors are, he said, at the very foundation of being alive and are, as such, essential expressions of human thinking. Therefore, in thinking about complex interactions of human systems, Bateson (Capra, 1988) offered the following syllogism that is based in metaphor in place of the commonly used one that is based in logic. In place of men die, Socrates dies, Socrates is a man, he offered men die, grass dies, men are grass. Freedom from fear of connection, complexity, and flexible organization are, indeed, three characteristic qualities of relational thinking. Bateson (Capra, 1988) is quoted as saying that he thought the more complicated the world became, the more beautiful it was.

Practitioners and researchers in family therapy wanted to experience firsthand the network of interpersonal relationships in a family rather than hear about them from individual family members one at a time. They wanted to experience directly the system in its complexity. This experience is similar to seeing a group, but very different, as well. Family members have a different order of emotional investment in one another and a history of shared experiences, triumphs, conflicts, losses, and treasured moments. Through projective processes, groups can mirror family strengths and unresolved issues. But the politics of a family can be very different from the politics of a newly formed group. Families, with their invested histories and family cultures, are powerful entities and can be intimidating to professionals working with them. Realizing that these families are, indeed, more powerful can be a relief and a safeguard in the process, as well. If the interventions do not fit or if their timing is not right, the family will push them back. Connecting or establishing working alliances with a whole group of family members is much different than working with an adult or even a dyad. The connection process thrusts the professional into the family's interpersonal and emotional space and can lead to visceral experiences of the pushes and pulls within it. Such experience is a clear indicator that actual connection is occurring and that the therapeutic system is forming. The professional begins to get empathic clues about what it is like to be in the family from the perspective of each of the members and confronts her own responses to these realities on the basis of her subjective perspective and history. Technical training and skill development, reflective practices, reflective supervision, and self-awareness development provide the tools necessary for navigation of the dynamic forces in a family system and catalyze the movement of family members toward jointly constructed, constructive goals of growth and healing. For family members, new experiences within old relationships and movement and change in real time within the therapy room create hope and build both motivation and momentum for cascading systemic changes. For professionals, live supervision behind a one-way mirror and invested self-awareness development processes in collegial groups provide indispensable collegial support and potential for growth.

Culture has something to do with fit of theoretical orientation for a professional. There are many different ways in which a professional can choose to ally with an orientation, but allying in some thoughtful way that has resonance and meaning contributes to a feeling of ease and fit with that orientation. For me, the focus on relationship and on the significance of emotional relationship contexts was very much in line with the perspective on life that I had gained from growing up in India. It made deep, intuitive sense; it mirrored my beliefs and expectations and gave me something that was familiar in a large body of individually oriented literature—literature that was fascinating and eye-opening but, nonetheless, left my cultural context out.

The view of a system of relationships applies to extended family and community as well as to larger systems such as the child welfare system, the preschool system, children's systems of care, the justice system, and so forth. It also extends to interdisciplinary relationships such as those between psychologists, family therapists, physicians, social workers, paraprofessional workers, nurses, and so forth. A system of relationships is a way of thinking. So, for example, little Elizabeth, who is in foster care with the plan of reunification with her mother, may be receiving monitored visits separately with her separated mother and father. Her mother, who has a bipolar diagnosis, receives individual therapy and medications management and has completed her required parenting classes. Her elderly father, who is 25 years her mother's senior, attends Alcoholics Anonymous. Elizabeth herself receives foster care services and in-home play therapy services as a way of helping her deal with all of the stressors and traumas that she has experienced in her young life. A foster family agency social worker and a county social worker coordinate the case, attend court, and work with the family toward eventual reunification. What a professional with a systemic orientation can naturally add to this array of services is case conceptualization and treatment planning that include linkages between services. Linkages, in this case, could be facilitation of constructive and potentially rich exchanges between biological and foster parents about changes, successes, struggles, and experiences (P. Minuchin, Colapinto, & Minuchin, 1998) with Elizabeth. They could discuss what she is like when she wakes up each morning, what her favorite foods are these days, how she responds to the outdoors or to her stroller, what her different cries mean, what some of her favorite gestures and words are. Or, perhaps, they could talk about what she was like as a baby, her most liked elements in her bedtime routine, what helped her rest, what made her fitful, what set her off, what soothed her the most, and what helped her recover. This communication between her multiple, serially separated caregivers can bridge the gaps between her psychological existences and holding in these relationships and can pave the way for a smoother eventual reunification. Further linkages prior to and following such reunification can provide family therapy support and guidance to the birth mother as she translates parenting class information into successful handling of the stresses in her actual situation of parenting her daughter and as she manages her mental health condition and medications. All too often, parents cannot make this bridge of connection between parenting class information and its application in actual interpersonal relationship contexts, especially in the face of stressors. Working directly with the family, in real time, on interpersonal relationship contexts can provide this help in a quality-of-life/cost-effective/time-effective way. In addition to providing such linkages to strengthen the family structure through communication, support, and guidance, the therapist can facilitate dyadic relational work by enhancing each parent's awareness of Elizabeth's emotional needs and responsiveness to them through observation, play, and interaction using models such as Bernstein's observations (Bernstein, Hans, & Percansky, 1991), Seeing Is Believing (Erickson,1999), and so forth. Numerous other evidence-based practices that focus on the parent–child relationship are also available for use (e.g., Cohen, Lojkasek, Muir, & Parker, 2002; Dozier, Higley, Albus, & Nutter, 2002; Lieberman, Silverman, & Pawl, 2000; Weider & Greenspan, 2005).

Systems thinkers are apt to focus on building bridges or linkages between the variety of services provided, conceptualize the links between the individual/dyadic/familial components of those services, and pass on to clients the ability to make such connections in their day-to-day lives. This can help parents consolidate learning from different services, understand how and why these services fit together, and prioritize attention to specific, present needs in the family. The experience of gaining such competence in the whole family context is like throwing a pebble into a pool: This pebble makes the first ripple and then progressively generates many others. It teaches a way of living and breathing in interconnected relational systems. As Milton Erickson (in Haley, 1973) said, the deviation-amplifying forces in a system make it possible for this to happen, for a small but significant systemic change to bring about many, many others. Similarly, in the words of Salvador Minuchin, family therapy is

an approach to treating human problems by bringing together the members of a family to help them work out conflicts at their source. But it also a new approach to understanding human behaviour as fundamentally shaped by its social context (S. Minuchin & Nichols, 1993, p. 35).

Structural Family Therapy

Minuchin created the structural family therapy model on the basis of his early clinical work (S. Minuchin, Montalvo, Guerney, Rosman, & Schumer, 1967). He saw the patterns in relationship systems, appreciated the importance of the relationship context in individual functioning, and acted on the need he saw in families for direct, organizing interventions. This need was particularly true in the underorganized families with whom he worked in New York City. The consolidation of his approach led to the form-/structure-/shape-focused structural model (S. Minuchin, 1974).

In structural family therapy, as in all systems work, individuals are viewed in a social context and, most especially, in their most intimate social context: the family, a network of socioemotionally significant relationships. The structure of this family is constituted by a set of relationships between family members and the rules governing them. The rules are influenced by culture—family culture as well as culture that is more broadly defined. Therefore, complex factors become implicated here, including individual and family life-cycle developmental stages, ethnicity, socioeconomic class, religion of family members, sexual orientation, gender balance, and power structure among members. These relationships and the rules that hold them together create the shape/structure of the family. Change is directed toward the structure of the group, which leads to changes in the position or role within the structure, which then leads to changes in subjective experiences and the nature of interactions and relationships between family members. An individually oriented professional looks at a phenomenon with a magnifying lens; a systems-oriented professional uses a zoom lens (S. Minuchin, 1974).

Joining is the structural therapy term for building an alliance or a trusting professional relationship. Although it shares much in common with these synonymous terms, the systemic implications of joining have certain nuances. These nuances illustrate that through the process of relationship building and directly experiencing the family relationships, the professional begins to integrate subjective and objective aspects of interpersonal process. This means, for example, that in patterns of behavior, patterns of responsivity, or nonresponsiveness of a caregiver to an infant, fine-tuned attunement or rough-hewn attunement are observed and experienced. It also means that the intrusiveness or responsivity and support of a grandmother in the family to the caregiver–infant dyad are observed and experienced repetitively. This experience provides the opportunity for an empathic basis of knowing what it may be like for the infant, caregiver, and grandmother to be in these relationships together, what is going well, what is in sync with cultural expectations, what is stressful, and what each person wants to see changed and preserved. On the basis of such an integrated understanding of subjective and objective sources of information, the professional can lead the family system catalytically in discussions of common goals, first steps, next steps, and strategies to achieve them. Identifying a family member's strengths in a similarly intimate way—that is, from an experienced and digested understanding of their particular strengths—is also very important in the joining process because it brings out the resiliencies and capacities that distressed and stressed families forget they have. Skill in pointing out something subtle but true, something that they may have forgotten, can be a profoundly connecting experience in itself and can help empower family members to engage in the process of needed or desired change. Minuchin used metaphors often and described joining as an experience that telescopes time and creates bonds of understanding between people. It is an element of the process that runs through the course of professional work, but in its initial stages, he described it as providing the anesthesia for later surgery. He has also called it the glue that holds the entire professional encounter together. Take your pick of metaphor!

Family maps are an ingenious and economical way of characterizing and representing family relationships and rules or the family structure. Through use of two structural dimensions, *boundaries* and *power structure/hierarchy,* family maps can be graphically drawn for purposes of assessment and goal setting. An excellent source for family maps is S. Minuchin (1974). The *power structure* refers to the authority or decision-making structure within the family and whether it is in sync with developmental (family and individual) and cultural expectations. *Boundaries* refer to several things. They mark roles within families and delineate subsystems or parts of families. Subsystems can be formed by gender (the female or male groups in the family), by interest (those who bowl, golf, or hike together), by generation (grandparents, parents, children), or by function (spousal or parental). They also describe the closeness–distance or preferred emotional styles of relating. These preferred emotional styles are depicted on a continuum from e*nmeshed/overinvolved/diffuse relationships* to *disengaged/underinvolved/rigid relationships*. *Enmeshment* refers to high-contact, high-intensity interactions, preference for closeness and proximity, emphasis on interdependence, and relationship/family or group goals. *Disengagement* refers to high independence, privacy, and preference for distance and individual goals. The terms, although they can sound somewhat dysfunctional, are thought to be so if they are held in the extreme, if they are held rigidly, and if they are accompanied by symptomatology. Cultural influences and individual histories affect these preferences—for example, cosleeping of infants and young children through the early years may be depicted as enmeshed but normal in a particular cultural context and not in another. This is similar for weaning and for acting autonomously (Carlson & Harwood, 2000). Only at the extremes on the continuum, when accompanied with identifiable symptomatology, can enmeshment or disengagement be termed dysfunctional. In the case of enmeshment, this may be if (a) parent–child enmeshment interferes with the perceptual–motor or affective–cognitive development of a young child or with the mastery of areas of development or if (b) strong contagion incapacitates family members coping under stress such that stress reverberates through the family and denudes its resiliencies. In the case of disengagement, this may take the form of a skewed sense of independence, lack of loyalty, or protectiveness shown toward family members in ordinary, everyday, culturally expected circumstances. Movement toward the increasing rigidity of preferred patterns, especially under stress, when these patterns may not be working, is indicative of systemic dysfunction. Flexibility and exploration of alternatives in such circumstances is an indication of functionality and well-being.

The assessment of family structure (hierarchy and boundaries in the context of family culture) provides the opportunity for giving family members feedback, engaging them in dialogue about goals, and jointly prioritizing these goals. This sets the stage for implementation of the goals, which entails relying on the quality of joining and the motivation and readiness of the family for change. Emphasizing strengths is a powerful way of continuing to build motivation and the courage to learn, grow, and change. *Enacting* typical challenging interactions, such as a negotiation between two parents regarding a disagreement about their infant's evening schedule, can be a very useful strategy. For example, in a family with two fathers, one parent wants to follow the baby's cues and put her to bed, and the other parent, who comes home later, misses the baby and wants to interact with her for a longer time before putting her to bed. The baby responds to the active parent, plays and enjoys the interaction for a while, and then gets cranky, gets overtired, and has a difficult time going to sleep. Both parents are frustrated by the end of this repeating routine. Enactment (or role playing, of a kind) brings such interactions, along with their flavor and context, back into the room. The professional can experience them firsthand, connecting with the way in which one father abruptly jumps into the fray and claims his right to playtime with his daughter, how she warms up to him and jumps right in, too, and also connecting with the way in which the other father, who, minutes earlier, was enjoying a quiet and pleasant time with his daughter, grows a little cold, quiet, and anxious. This parent goes along with it, makes room for the play, and, later, joins in as a threesome. But the anxiety in him remains for the rest of the time, the slightly resentful anxiety of a sensitive parent who has not been heard in the interactions. The clinician experiences all of this empathically and intervenes, asking the anxious parent what he might like to say; he backs off, and the other parent leaps in, saying that the anxious parent just does not like his style of play in the evenings. The clinician is puzzled and asks if the couple wants the child to have two parents or only one at a time? The couple is puzzled, the active father more so than the withdrawing one. The clinician asks the withdrawing one if the question makes sense. He nods and offers that when the two of them are together, his partner takes over all the decisions, all the answering, and he (the withdrawing one) steps back. The clinician nods affirmatively and asks the parents if they want it this way. Their silence speaks, as do their facial expressions. They are in a quandary. The clinician challenges the quandary by asking how they want things to change. They say that they do not like how their interactions feel, but they do not know how to make them different. The clinician wonders if the idea of space in critical places would help—that is, if the active father could create some space between his desire to play with his daughter and his acting on that desire enough to take a breath, talk, and connect with his partner first. The clinician wonders if the withdrawing father could create some space between his attunement to his daughter's daily rhythm and his backing off in the face of his partner's lack of attunement to it enough to stop himself from disappearing in the conversation. They listen with sensitivity and interest. The suggestion makes sense, and they are encouraged to take deep breaths, slow down, and reenact with these suggestions. They talk with one another; the active parent leads, asking about his partner's day and his daughter's early evening. His partner responds warmly, explaining that her nanny said that she really enjoyed the park. The withdrawing father says that he knows her eyes glow when she sees the active father but that the withdrawing father needs him to understand that it is the end of her day and she is tired. They hear one another and play gently with their daughter. Use of the experiential component in empathic and skilled ways gives the fathers a holding and guiding environment in which they can work on their dilemma as they find new awarenesses and ways of communicating to work through their impasses with one another.

Intensity raising is an intervention of which Minuchin is a master, and many of his professional tapes demonstrate it well. He describes intensity as stroking and kicking, nurturing and challenging to unbalance the system, to shake it up enough so that it can flexibly and, on its own, reorganize as natural systems are apt to do. Such action can be taken profitably when the joining with the family is strong and dependable. For example, consider the case of an Indian American family in which a young couple is preparing to formalize the name of their infant child in a traditional naming ceremony. Both parents are professional and well-educated, and so are their extended families. They have engaged in active conversation with one another and with their extended families and friends on both sides about a possible name. They have bought books about naming a child that provide traditional and contemporary Indian names from various ethnic and religious and communities, explaining etymological roots and meanings. The couple creates a short list with help from the extended network. No name has been chosen yet. However, as the time for the ceremony draws close, the paternal grandfather steps forward and declares proudly that he has chosen the formal name for his grandson. The child's father appears mildly ambivalent but is willing to appease his father and go along with it, but the mother is not at all willing to do so; therefore, the couple is in conflict. The clinician raises intensity with the couple by saying that he is confused because it seems as though they are taking two opposite roads at the same time. He asks if they, as a couple, shared patriarchical or egalitarian beliefs. He observes that they started off very collaboratively and then, very abruptly, the process became hierarchical and traditional. He asks where they stand.

The husband says that he is confused: He wants to be collaborative and he believes in him and his wife having equal voices, but he does not know how to stand up to his father or to a very old legacy of male privilege and tradition within his family. He also does not want to hurt the feelings of his elderly father, who is not confused at all about this and believes in male privilege. The wife is touched by her husband's opening up and says that she, too, does not want to hurt her father-in-law's feelings. She wonders if her husband could speak with his father about their feelings. She says that her father-in-law is an affectionate and caring man who is not aware that their feelings were being hurt in this process. With the neutralizing of some of the conflict and anxiety through the collaborative, supportive discussion, the husband agrees to speak with his father. They speak man to man, and his father acknowledges his pride in the couple and his desire to not hurt them in any way. Uplifted by his emotional connection and conversation with his father, the son works out a strategy enabling his father to be an important part of, but not the final say on, the name. He asks his father to look over their list of names and to identify a short list of names that resonate with him. The father does, and then the son and his wife choose the final name from this short list. Thus, through the use of intensity raising, family conflict is neutralized and culturally in-sync family development is facilitated. For the infant, his formal name and the processes through which it is chosen provide a strong, positive, culturally grounded foundation in family relationships with important meanings, bases for sociocultural identity, and resiliencies that he will discover as he grows older. The family maps capturing the clinician's work with this family system are depicted in Figure 2.2.

Figure 2.2 Assessment and goal setting maps.

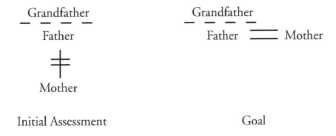

Initial Assessment   Goal

Spatial repositioning, or paying attention to closeness–distance information and cultural meanings in the way people sit, stand, or move vis a vis one another and suggesting alternatives, is another way of changing people's experience of their family structure. Engaging family members in the exploration of this change is a simple but incredibly powerful way of restructuring systems and can be a first step toward engaging them in dialogue. Minuchin speaks of spatial positioning as having graphic eloquence; indeed, moving family members vis a vis one another with a grasp of their underlying structure and in line with their cultures and stated goals can be far more powerful than words and can open up new possibilities in relationships and new discussions about them.

Structural Questions: Suggestions for Clinicians

1. *What is the joining process with the family like?*

2. *What are the family's strengths?*

3. *How would you characterize the family structure (hierarchy and boundaries) in this family's cultural context?*

4. *How would you represent the family structure on a family map?*

5. *What are the prioritized, culturally in-sync goals for restructuring the family?*

6. *What restructuring interventions will you use to achieve these goals?*

7. *What aspects of personal experience (connection, culture, countertransference) do you want to be especially attentive to in restructuring the family?*

Strategic Family Therapy

Close on the heels of the structural model came the strategic one by Jay Haley (Haley, 1987; Haley & Richeport-Haley, 2003). He coined the term *strategic family therapy* to define a type of therapy in which the clinician initiates what happens in treatment and designs an individualized approach for each problem (Haley, 1987). Here again, Greenspan's (Greenspan & Benderly, 1997) emphasis on the individuality of development finds a mirror in the context of mental health treatment. Professional work in human science and human service can hardly afford to be unfamiliar with or isolating of the richness of subjective experience. In so being, it dooms us to an utter incompleteness of knowledge that we may not seek or to which we may not aspire.

The strategic model is very similar to the structural one. Haley is the ultimate pragmatist, however, and presents a model of action, adamant that insight is neither needed nor sought in the change process. I have found that there are at least as many people who care about insight as there are not, but people in distress, whoever they are, generally want help with solving their problems. I have also found, in my clinical experience, that although insight may not be a prerequisite or preferred route to change for everyone, it can actually follow the experience of change just as it can precede it. Haley presents other odd notions about therapy. For example, Haley asserts that if one leaves out culture and the complexity of culture, one can be briefer, and being brief and having the ability to problem solve are the hallmarks of strategic therapy. However, in Haley's work in other cultural contexts, such as among the shamans of Bali in Indonesia, the parallels that he draws from Zen philosophy in his work seem to indicate that the essence of culture and cultural understanding are very much present at the heart of his work, though he claims it is bereft of it! The strategies of Haley's model have proven very useful over time in work with parents and children.

Strategic family therapy has one central point of difference from the structural one and has other finer points of variation. Its focus is on the process of interactions around the presenting problem in place of the overall family structure. The *presenting problem* is stated and agreed upon in very clear, concrete, and definable terms. If there is more than one presenting problem, the family will be engaged in a process of prioritizing those problems. The *interpersonal sequences of interactions* through which the presenting problem plays itself out—that is, who does what, when and how is it done, how does it end, when does it happen or not happen, how often does it happen, are there variations on a theme, and so forth—are mapped out through the tracking process in early family interviews. The presenting problem, demonstrated through repetitive interaction patterns called *sequences of interaction*, are clearly identified.

Family organization or structure is also looked at, but the approach, or lens, is to start with the microcosm of family process that typifies the presenting problem and sequences of interaction between the family members and to see these sequences in the context of the family structure. In the structural approach, one strives to understand the family structure first and identifies the ways in which the problem represents a problem in the structure. Two elements of the hierarchy are points of interest in the strategic model. The first is that the hierarchy be in line with the values, beliefs, expectations, or culture of the family; the second is whether there are corruptions of hierarchy such as rigid, cross-generational coalitions. Every family, no matter what their culture, makes an elemental hierarchical distinction between parents and young children. *Cross-generational coalitions,* or a repeated, rigid parent–child emotional alliance that leaves out the other parent or members of the family's executive system, is clinically observed to be indicative of dysfunction. In the strategic model, the emphasis is on identification of these two elements of family structure. On the matter of the family hierarchy functioning in sync with cultural values, consider the example of a Japanese American family who has two homes—a main house and a guest house—on a single property. A young couple and their new child live in the main house. The father's parents live in another town in the same state, and they visit often. When they do, they live in the guest house. The older generation is *nisei,* or second generation, in the United States; their son is *sansei,* or third generation; and his wife is a first-generation immigrant from Japan. The day-to-day decisions in the young family's life are made by them, but major decisions regarding rites of passage and other family issues, financial issues, and so forth, are made jointly by the older couple and the younger couple, with the father and grandfather playing a patriarchical role of ultimate authority in the process. In contrast to this is the example of a Caucasian American woman living alone with her young son. She is fifth-generation American with Polish, Italian, and Irish ancestry, and she has been recently widowed. Her mother, also a widow, lives a few streets away in the same neighborhood. The two women meet and connect daily, enjoy a close relationship, and handle their life decisions relatively independently but lean on one another to air their thoughts and to be one another's sounding board. The younger woman states that if her husband had been alive, she likely would have been somewhat more distant with her mother in regards to various decision-making issues, relying on her husband more, but she still would have talked and shared information with her mother and would have been available for her in the same way as she is now. Both young children in both families are learning, through their socialization processes, about hierarchy within their families. However, their experiences vary with the cultures, beliefs, and circumstances of their families. Figure 2.3 depicts these different but culturally normative family hierarchies in each of the two families.

Family life-cycle stages emphasized by Erickson (Haley, 1973) and written about extensively by Carter and McGoldrick (2005) is another contextual yardstick used in the strategic approach. The stages of becoming a couple and forming a family, or choosing to have a baby by nontraditional means or without becoming a couple (stage A), having a new baby (stage B), or becoming a family with multiple children (stage C) are family life-cycle stages relevant to multicultural infant–family

Figure 2.3 Cultural variation in normative family structure.

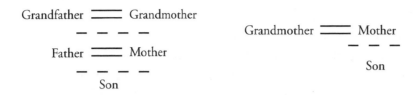

mental health. Family life-cycle transitions bring with them new psychosocial tasks, and their timing and nature are dictated by culture (family culture and broader culture). Carter and McGoldrick provide some guidelines that are presented and elaborated upon here. In stage A, the family psychosocial tasks include committing to a new family system through forming a couples system and realigning relationships with extended family, friends, and community to include partner/spouse. This new family may be a nuclear entity or may be part of a loosely or tightly defined, extended-family entity. In stages B and C, the family psychosocial tasks include accepting new members into the family, which family members express by adjusting the couples system to make space for a child/children; sharing child rearing, financial, and household tasks; and realigning relationships with extended family and friends to include parents, grandparents, godparents, and other supportive coparenting roles (e.g., aunts/uncles) in extended families. In stage C, the facilitation of sibling relationships—for example, relationships between older children and newly arrived infants as well as relationships with cousins and peers (e.g., playgroup/preschool)—and attention to the individual development and needs of each child become relevant.

In families in which children's ages are spaced out, especially in blended families, other family life-cycle stages may be relevant, such as in families with both adolescents (stage D) and infants/toddlers. In this case, the family psychosocial tasks of stages B and C come into play along with the additional tasks of stage D, which are increasing the flexibility of family boundaries to include the adolescent's independence and the grandparents' frailty. This stage may be expressed in several ways: Parents making space for adolescents and later curfews; adolescents driving, holding jobs, and so forth; and roles for making additional family contributions (e.g., babysitting), facilitating sibling relationships, negotiating family loyalty and sibling rivalry issues, maintaining attention to the needs of individual children, refocusing midlife couples and career issues, and addressing caring for older generations. In families in which grandparents (stage E) become foster or adoptive parents of infants and toddlers, the psychosocial tasks of stages B and C, and the tasks of stage E, come into play. Stage E can include launching older children and/or grandchildren; accepting these exits and entries into the family system; renegotiating shared parenting issues in light of physical/and or financial decline; balancing community engagements, resources, and supports with parenting needs; and making room for wisdom, experience, and meaning to support family and community relationships.

In addition to these numerous and complex family psychosocial life-cycle tasks, there are individual psychosocial life-cycle tasks of (a) establishing trust (in place of distrust) in infancy and (b) establishing autonomy and initiative (in place of shame, doubt, and guilt) in toddlerhood (Erikson, 1963). Parents' individual psychosocial tasks can range from establishing intimacy (in place of isolation), role flexibility (in place of role rigidity), social relatedness (in place of social withdrawal), and generativity (in place of stagnation), depending on the age and situation of a parent or a parenting grandparent.

Clearly, family life-cycle and individual life-cycle psychosocial tasks are multiple and complex in the life of any family with a young child and can, themselves, be sources of stress. Awareness and knowledge of them offer sources of clarity, meaning, direction, and support. A clinician's awareness of these psychosocial tasks can be useful in assessing the presenting problems in the context of these tasks and in intervening with families to engage them in dialogue on the specific psychosocial tasks relevant to their life situation. Generating new ways of looking at, coping with, and negotiating these tasks can become an empowering experience in therapy. In addition, clinician sensitivity and awareness of life-cycle transitions can facilitate empathic connection with families and help normalize the stress of life-cycle transitions.

The working method in the strategic approach is the creation of direct or indirect (paradoxical) directives. The former are addressed here only as they seem particularly relevant in multicultural infant–family mental health. *Directives* are interventions in which the particular sequences of interactions through which the presenting problem is lived out over and over again are interrupted and alternative sequences are offered with motivating rationales to the family. The professional must understand all of the information regarding the working relationship, structure, and culture to come up with suggestions of alternative action—suggestions that change family interaction patterns around the presenting problems and shift them in the direction of stated goals. Thus, connection with the family members and their unique process as well as imagination, ingenuity, and creativity are involved in coming up with individualized directives session after session until problems are successively solved.

To give an example of the strategic model, we turn to Joe, the young son of Caucasian American parents who was "fighting too much" with peers at his day care. He was nearly 3 and was very bright, expressive, active, and well-coordinated. Joe was the apple of his mother's eye, her first and only child. She was devoted to his care, and she delighted in him. She worked as a secretary and receptionist and looked forward to her family time in the evenings and on the weekends. An energetic and outgoing person, the mother was the one most concerned with her son's behavior, and she sought help. The father was soft spoken and mild mannered. He had an assembly line job and worked long hours. He, too, was devoted to his family and enjoyed being home with them; he had a quiet presence, generally, but was roused into roughhousing by his son from time to time. The mother generally took Joe to the day care and was the one who heard the complaints about the fighting. These fights happened at least three or four times a week and sometimes more. The teachers reported that the fights seemed to come out of nowhere. They were not about sharing or about some action by another child that he did not like. Joe seemed to intrude into a child's space or body, and he did so before anyone knew there would be a fight. It sounded a lot like roughhousing going awry.

Working strategically, the clinician accepted the parents' definition of the presenting problem of "too much fighting," thus affirming their executive authority in the family and aligning herself with them. The sequences of interaction around this presenting problem were that Joe would jump on another boy's body or into his play space unexpectedly, the peer would push him back or shove him, and they would begin to fight. The teacher would break them up, would say to Joe that he must not start fights, and would give him a time out, which he would take quietly; then, he would resume his activities. The mother would pick up Joe and receive a slip of paper on which the fighting incident would be reported. She would feel upset about the occurrence; talk with the teacher; and assure her that she talks with Joe about this, would continue to do so, and would return home with him. She would remind Joe not to fight at school and that it is not a good way to make friends, and she would talk with her husband about her concerns. Her husband would listen but usually would not offer any perspectives, and he would not deal directly with Joe on the matter, either.

A motivating rationale for the family was (a) validation of the parents' concern and commitment to help their son by coming together to work on it and (b) the importance of continuing to work together for his sake. In addition, it was elaborated that Joe was moving into a time in his life when he was discovering that he was a boy and that he needed closeness with his father. With this rationale, a directive was given to head off a potential cross-generational coalition between Joe and his mother against his father, and an intermediate coalition was set up between Joe and his father. It was requested that his father pick him up from day care and spend more time with him, especially around his problem behavior, finding out from the teacher and from Joe what was happening and responding to it. His father was amenable to this request, and Joe's mother made room for his father to step in. Joe's father said that he could do this every day except one day in the week when his schedule did not permit it. So, it was arranged that his mother would stand in on that day. In the coming weeks, Joe's problem behavior began to lessen in frequency, and in 3 weeks, it was virtually a nonissue. His father was willing and happy to be more involved in Joe's care, and his mother was able to make more room for Joe's father but was getting anxious in her unfamiliar, off-center position. To alleviate the mother's anxiety, the clinician gave her a directive in the following way. Observing that she was an expert in dealing with people, as her work required it, and that she had previously reported that she enjoyed that work and did it well, the clinician gave the mother the job of creating three 20-minute special times for her and Joe. In these activities, they would play and pretend they were in day care, and she would show him various good ways of making friends and expressing feelings of being mad. She was excited at the idea, keen to be engaged with Joe in this way, so she took the directive. Joe's progress continued, and follow-up sessions were suggested in accordance with the strategic model. These sessions were scheduled for 1 month, 3 months, and 6 months later. In the follow-up sessions, it was found that Joe and his family had moved on from the problem of "fighting too much." Both parents were enjoying their connections with him, and he was a much happier child for the balanced, daily access that he felt he had to both of them.

The sequences of interaction maintained and provided a window into Joe's experience with a bonded mother who, nonetheless, gave Joe's father very little room in the parenting relationship. His father—who was himself mild mannered, distant, and of the cultural mindset that parenting was mostly his wife's work and that his wife was very good at it—did not take it upon himself to redress the balance in any way. When, on occasion, Joe had a chance to roughhouse with his father, Joe felt really close and connected, and he liked that. At the time of the fighting, Joe had been becoming more aware of his gender identity as a boy and was missing this connection with his father in his life. Thus, he acted out upon his peers a common way in which children can speak their needs and distresses. The *intermediate coalition* that was created when the clinician gave the job of handling Joe's problems to his father brought his father closer to him. The task of *clearing/balancing the hierarchy,* which the clinician facilitated by assigning Joe's mother the job of helping him express angry feelings and creatively problem solve in peer relationships (by taking turns, sharing, getting help, etc.), gave the mother and father equal but different connections to him around his present psychological challenges. This approach gave them the experience as well as a model that demonstrated a way to be engaged together with Joe in other areas on other issues. The family maps in Figure 2.4 graphically depict these shifts in family dynamics.

Figure 2.4 Assessment, intermediate, and final goal maps.

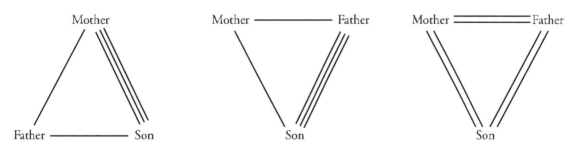

The family had weathered the previous life-cycle stage of being a family with a new child, Joe, in infancy and early toddlerhood. At this stage, Joe was very closely tied to his mother and less so to his father. As Joe was growing older, his family remained stuck on this pattern, and it was not serving his developmental needs very well. Even in the voice of symptoms we can hear the desire of the human being to be healthy and whole, as we hear in Joe's symptoms the need for identification with his father and balanced connections with both parents.

Strategic Questions: Suggestions for Clinicians

1. *What is the presenting problem?*

2. *What are the interpersonal sequences of interaction around the problem?*

3. *Is the family hierarchy functional and in sync with the family's culture and values?*

4. *Are there any fixed/rigid cross-generational coalitions in this family?*

5. *What is this family's life-cycle or developmental stage?*

6. *What directive and motivating rationale can you offer the family to change the presenting problem?*

7. *What is noteworthy in reflecting on your experience as a clinician with this family as you work on these steps with them?*

Paradoxical Family Therapy

There are several approaches to paradoxical family therapy. Those approaches offered by the Mental Research Institute (MRI) of Palo Alto, California, and the Milan School of Italy are integrated here and are offered as two representative samples of paradoxical therapy. In a small but influential book called *Change: Principles of Problem Formation and Problem Resolution,* Paul Watzlawick and colleagues (Watzlawick, Weakland, & Fisch, 1974) described the MRI approach to homeostasis/stability and change in family systems. Symptoms develop when families face a challenge that they address with tried-and-true methods, even if these methods are not solving the particular problem at hand. They might persist with the same solutions despite the lack of encouraging results and, therefore, the *interactional solutions* that they use may, themselves, become the problem. In this way, an original challenge or difficulty, along with the family's interactional solutions, can become entrenched in the system as a problem or symptom. The authors looked deeply at the nature of systemic change and stability and distinguished between *first-order changes,* or minor changes within existing frameworks, and *second-order changes,* or major changes that involve discontinuous leaps between frameworks, taking systems into states of greater complexity. The authors were more concerned with the second type of change—major, sudden, unexpected change that is halting of logic and breaking of tempo. In this sense, they, too, were Zen-like in their inclinations and in their techniques, posing paradoxical solutions to systemic arrests to engage the family system in its own positive growth.

In MRI, the authors analogically used a mathematical theory called the *theory of groups* to illustrate the features of stability. This theory points to four factors that keep things the same or stable: (a) having a *common denominator,* or something in the group that all family members have in common that binds them; (b) moving within an agreed upon framework of rules and understandings; (c) having a *group preserver,* or someone or some subset of the group who is strongly invested in the status quo, and (d) using an opposites strategy that cancels out the possibility of change from either one. In families in which first-order changes are needed and none are being applied, these stabilizing factors are useful to consider. They can provide needed stability. In families in which second-order changes are needed and first-order changes are being used, these stabilizers are also useful to consider, because they can be barriers to needed growth and change.

A family's first-order solutions are categorized by MRI as falling into four different categories. These categories are, first, interactional solutions that involve actions that are *more of the same,* or *wrong, action* (such as Joe's mother's overinvolved and ineffective interactions with him around fighting with peers); *inaction* (such as Joe's father's standing-back behavior); or *action where unnecessary* (e.g., action resulting from lack of acceptance of diversity, generational differences, and other differences that need to be understood and accepted rather than changed). The second category is interactional solutions that involve perception, such as *simplification,* in which there are problems of denial of vulnerability (grandiosity) or of competence (low self-esteem). The third category is another type of interactional solution that also involves perception—*utopian* or unrealistic solutions. The fourth category is interactional solutions of action and perception that are *paradoxical,* self-reflexive, and contradictory, such as saying one thing and doing the opposite or saying one thing in words and saying its opposite in tone of voice, gesture, or facial expression, such as in double-binding communications (Banerjee & Roy, 1987; Banerjee & Sawyers, 1986; Banerjee & Sawyers, 1990).

The Milan group (Palazolli, Boscolo, Cecchin, & Prata, 1975/1978) uses the idea of a *family rule* to articulate a family's governance and stability. In times of distress in dysfunctioning families, inflexible family rules and endless, innovative variations of fundamentally the same inflexible family rules are implicated. For example, Patricia is 30 years of age, Hispanic American, and divorced for a year and a half from her husband Victor, who is 32 years of age. She lives with their 3-year-old son Jose in her parents' home. Both of Jose's parents work and share legal custody, and Jose attends a small family day care program. Both parents subscribe to strong pro-family cultural values. Jose sees his father on weekends but has difficulty leaving his mother, both at day care and on the weekends, although less so on the weekends. He has had his day care arrangement for more than 6 months, and his separation continues to be a difficult issue. Jose sleeps in a separate bed in his mother's room and in his father's room on weekends. He has started having disturbed night sleep as well, waking, at times, from crying or restlessness. He is progressing well, developmentally, and generally is a cheerful child when he is in the presence of his mother.

What could we be hearing about a family rule in this family through the voice of the child, keeping in mind that caregiver affect and the affective climate of family relationships influence the child? Family interviews revealed that the family fears or is very ambivalent about separation. Jose's father holds on to the fantasy that his mother will reconcile with him and that the family will reunite. His mother fears that if she allows her son to grow up, he will become independent and leave her. Jose acts out both his parents' and his own fearfulness. As a child of divorce, he may have fears of losing both his parents and/or fears of being guilty of causing the same. The rule in this family may be articulated in the following way: It is not safe to separate or to grow up because, in doing so, someone or something very important will be lost.

The Milan team developed the tool known as *circular questions* to get at the systemic information that creates awareness of family rules by asking family members to take turns in reflecting on the relationships of other members, and listening to such reflections. Five categories of these questions are asked of each family member, and, through the professional facilitation of dialogue, consensus on them is reached. This, itself, can be a substantial part of the work. The categories of the questions are about the problem, the sequences of interaction around the problem, the family structure (hierarchy, alliances, coalitions), the goals and change expected through the process, and, most important, the consequences of change. This last category of questions asks what the family would be left with if their problem fell away. The questions in this category seek answers beyond a simple "everything will be fine." They ask what the family would be faced with and would need to change if the problem itself were dissolved. Thus, these questions are very important in their potential to reveal the systemic function of the problem and the systemic resistance to change.

Analysis of *original difficulties* that families confront, analysis of the *stabilizers* in the form of interactional solutions that they use, and analysis of the family rules that govern their family relationships provide glimpses into the family's homeostasis and opportunities for empathic understanding of it. As empathic understanding of the family's idiosyncratic, emotional logic in the face of distress (at the cost of symptomatology) emerges for the clinician, these same interactional solutions or family rules can be positively restated to the family. This is the paradoxical intervention, variously known as *prescribing the problem, positive connotation,* or *paradoxical prescription,* which can be given verbally or in the form of a letter.

Paradoxical interventions are particularly useful in addressing long-standing, repetitious problems in which families exhibit strong ambivalence or opposition to change. These interventions are contraindicated in any type of situation in which safety issues are involved and in situations that call for structuring or crisis intervention types of measures. In situations in which resistance to change is high, the effective use of paradox, which aligns with the resistance, can bypass it and free the system to reorganize into a more complex, flexible system. Such a family system becomes capable and ready to

Family Systems and Culture

use untried strategies, new information, and developmentally fitting methods. The conceptual approaches of MRI and Milan are helpful in considering the symptom and the system of interactions (or sequences of interaction) and in connecting them with their meaning or function in the family system. This approach opens up the route to empathy between the professional and the family members, the route through which meaning can be offered in deeply insightful, systemic, paradoxical interventions. Being understood in respectful and meaningful ways, irrationalities and all, frees family members who are locked in oppositional dynamics from needing to pursue oppositional means to be heard. Being heard relieves tensions, builds connections, and allows the natural exploration of new alternatives.

In the case of Jose's family, this paradoxical intervention may take a form such as the following. His parents may be offered a letter that goes something like this:

> *You have both lost a great deal that has meaning for you, and you both are holding on to dearly held hopes to make it through. Above all, you have a precious child who you will always be parents of and whom you will always love. This, too, you have in common. But both of you are afraid, just as Jose is afraid. He feels so afraid inside now that he fears losing more at every turn, and day-to-day events such as separating from his mother or going to sleep at night remind him of this fear. You can understand that fear because each of you feels it too and, because of it, you (father) hold on to the precious hope of being reunited with your ex-spouse and you (mother) hold onto the impossible image of Jose being a small child forever. None of you want anymore change; it has been too much, and it has been too painful. Facing these losses and changes and their finality may be much, much more painful. Therefore, you find it is preferable and wiser to face the easier problem of Jose's fears. It is easier for him, too. Until both of you are ready and confident to face the bigger losses and pain that have touched and shaken your lives, you may decide to hold on to the smaller ones."*

A paradoxical intervention breaks free its recipients from the stranglehold of patterns they feel trapped in by making the covert overt. The family can no longer continue as before. They now have the choice to continue what they have been doing but with new awareness, meaning, and the benefit of being heard respectfully, deeply, and with acceptance. Or they can take the chance of tackling the bigger issues and making more radical second-order change, which will transform them and move them to the next evolutionary step in family development.

Paradoxical Questions: Suggestions for Clinicians

1. What was the original difficulty that the family was facing?

2. What are the stabilizing factors in this family?

3. What interactional solutions were used by the family?

4. What family rules are operative in this family?

5. How can you connote the function of the symptoms and these systems of interaction in a positive, deeply empathic, culturally connected, useful way?

6. Would you prefer to say or write the paradoxical intervention? If you write it will you give it to the family in person or mail them a copy?

7. How does your self as clinician speak to you and impact you in putting together this intervention?

Bowenian Family Therapy

Murray Bowen's (1985) work came from a pairing of observations in biology and psychiatry, and he offered a systemic model that covered interpersonal space as well as intrapersonal space, present-day interactions as well as historical, intergenerational interactions. He encapsulated these dimensions in the concept of *differentiation*. This concept represents socioemotional functioning in a continuum ranging from *fusion* to *cutoff*. Differentiation has an internal and an interpersonal dimension. Internally, it involves striking a balance between the drive and intensity of passion and the organization and structure of reason. Interpersonally, it involves striking a balance between connectedness with oneself and with others and loss of connection, be it by invasive or disengaging means. Differentiation, in other words, is about balance and connection with the interior of oneself and in relationships with others. This balance and connection lets a person direct his or her life in a way that is authentic for him or her and have relationships with people and things in a way that is authentic, as well. Similar to the work in attachment, the work in differentiation needs to be expanded through the inclusion of culture. The concept of differentiation itself is flexible, complex, and wide open for such accommodation, defined as it is by balance and connection in the interior and exterior of socioemotional life. However, a western bias in the differentiation literature is prevalent. Differentiation is interpreted as balance that leans toward autonomy/independence. This leaning may fit an individual and family and the legacy of a newborn in a particular instance, but in another instance, a balance that leans toward interdependence, or closer ties to ones' own needs in connection with those of others, may be more relevant (Chien & Banerjee, 2002). This difference also can be stated as the cultural and personal destiny of a newborn sapling either to be its own fir tree in a clearing of fir trees (independence orientation) or to be a new branch of an extensive Banyan tree (interdependence orientation; Chien & Banerjee, 2002). As discussed in the

Circle Two section on attachment, autonomy in an independence-focused culture can appear active and assertive, whereas in an interdependence-focused culture it can appear calm and receptive (Rothbaum & Morelli, 2005). Such diversity in the appearance of autonomy as it relates to differentiation is necessary to explore in clinical applications, measurement tools, and research. The diversity of our society and the diversity in our interconnected globe makes it not only imperative to expand our awareness and conceptualization in such ways but also motivating to do so.

Triangulation, or pulling third parties into the relationship of any two, occurs when levels of differentiation are low, whether it is expressed as fusion or as cutoff. When anxiety rises in the interactions between two people and when resiliencies and coping mechanisms are perceived as decreasing, triangulation provides welcome relief and lets the stress diffuse. But it also prevents the emergence of the kind of problem solving, dialogue, and understanding that can, more fundamentally, lower anxiety and can increase the level of differentiation. Thus, the higher the level of differentiation in a person or a relationship, the lower the need for triangulation.

Bowen's concept of fusion and Minuchin's concept of enmeshment as well as Bowen's concept of cutoff and Minuchin's concept of disengagement have some overlap. They are similar concepts in the context of interpersonal functioning. However, the Bowenian concept of differentiation underlies enmeshment–disengagement and provides the historical motivating force rooted in intergenerational family history for the expression of these relationship patterns. In the middle ranges of both concepts, there is less vacillation in connection or affiliation than there is at either extreme (Johnson & Waldo, 1998). Higher differentiation is related to four factors: (a) less emotional reactivity and greater calmness in response to stress or emotionality of others; (b) ability to take I-positions even under pressure; (c) freedom from fusion with others, demonstrated by freedom from need for acceptance and approval at all costs and above all else; and (d) freedom from cutoff, the capacity to stay connected under profoundly threatening circumstances without resorting to retreating into facades of independence through cutoff. Higher levels of differentiation are related to lower levels of chronic anxiety, better psychological adjustment, and lower levels of physical and psychological symptoms (Bowen, 1985; Kerr & Bowen, 1988; Titelman, 1998). The Differentiation of Self Inventory–Revised (Skowron & Schmidtt, 2003) facilitates the measurement of differentiation levels in adults through the assessment of these four factors. The differentiation in functioning of family members in present time is captured through the concept of the *nuclear family emotional process*. The transmission of differentiation level, unresolved issues, and resiliencies is captured by the concept of *multigenerational family projection process*.

Change occurs through connection with, and lowering of, the level of chronic anxiety within individuals in key relationships and family systems seen in a historical perspective. The tool used for this work is the *multigenerational family genogram*, which is used for observation, reflection, and experiential connection with this material with supportive holding, challenging, and coaching from a clinician. For professionals, the process of going back home—or, in other words, ongoing engagement with their own family and cultural history through a genogram—is not only a necessity but an empowering treasure trove of experience that can help the professional authentically and confidently lead others in the process (Aponte, 1994; Banerjee, 2000; Banerjee & Willingham, 1998; Hardy & Lazloffy, 1995). Stories, films, and exposure to genograms of others—as well as multiple family group therapy using genograms in which families can learn from one another and support one another in the process—can be facilitative of this journey.

Monica McGoldrick and colleagues (McGoldrick, Gerson, & Shellenberger, 1999) have produced a large body of work on genograms, laying out guidelines for conducting family interviews with questions for each section and stage and guidelines for gathering data from the family so that the family can place themselves in sociocultural/political/historical reality. The categories of questions that the authors provide and their clinical demonstrations, which are available in audiovisual formats (McGoldrick et al., 1999), are very helpful in orienting oneself to the work. These categories of questions include details about the presenting problem, questions on household context, information on the parents' birth families, questions about significant historical events across generations in family history, probing of cultural variables, questions about attitudes toward gender, details about major life events in the current family, questions about the nature of current relationships and family roles, and questions about the nature of individual functioning and goals. Repetitive family patterns and levels of differentiation are reflected upon jointly; coincidences, critical events and symptoms, losses and changes, untimely and timely family life-cycle transitions, and particular family traumas (McGoldrick et al., 1999) and resiliencies (Banerjee, 2000) are discussed and, thus, brought into awareness, connected with, and reflected upon. This process builds the family's capacity to increase emotional tolerance of intense anxieties, experience a wider range of emotions, and experience emotional regulation. It lowers chronic anxiety and emotional reactivity.

For example, Lucy, an Armenian American, is working in dyadic therapy as a way of attuning to her 2½-year-old son Fernando, from whom she was, earlier, quite disengaged. In the supportive context of dyadic therapy, in which the clinician is working with the dyadic relationship of mother and child, Lucy is able to distinguish how responsive Fernando is to her physical holding, touch, and soothing words when he is upset and how he feels that these same behaviors are intrusive when he is playing. As her connection and sensitivity to him is growing, she mentions that her son's biological father has recently reconnected with him and expressed his love for him. Lucy has noticed that this change in the status of Fernando's relationship with his father has calmed him considerably. She also states that she does not want to tell her parents about these events, positive though they may be. She lives with her parents and, so, is closely involved with them day to day. Her clinician wonders aloud if Lucy is concerned that her parents may not trust her to handle the situation well, which is a comment on the nuclear family emotional process. Lucy states that the clinician's empathy accurately reflects her struggle and reflects some culturally and generationally based differences in beliefs and expectations between her and her parents. It also reflects the type of fusion that exists between her as an adult daughter and her parents. She thinks that they will not trust her, that they will give her unwanted advice on how to handle her ex-husband, and that she will feel hurt and unsupported. There inevitably will be conflict that will bring up older conflicts, and it will be very stressful and will remain unresolved. Furthermore, Fernando will get stressed by all of this conflict. The clinician suggests that Lucy explore her autonomy struggles with her parents in intergenerational context through a genogram, as this struggle relates directly to her capacity to effectively facilitate Fernando's autonomy at a stage in life when this is coming to the fore for him. Lucy understands the rationale and, relying on the trusting relationship and professional competence of her clinician, enthusiastically enters the genogram process.

Bowenian Questions: Suggestions for Clinicians

1. *How would you describe the family's level of differentiation in a culturally in-sync way on the fusion-to-cutoff continuum?*

2. *What is the nuclear family's emotional process like as seen through its cultural lens?*

3. *How would you characterize the culturally influenced multigenerational transmission process of differentiation in this family?*

4. *What categories of questions and what specific questions would you use to guide the family through their genogram-drawing process?*

5. *What repetitive patterns, coincidences, and significant events are most pertinent in the life of this young child and his caregivers at the present time? How do these patterns, coincidences, and significant events empower the caregivers, and what areas need the support and facilitative process of intervention?*

Conclusion

Research provides strong evidence from longitudinal and other sources for family-based interventions in problems of early childhood (Boyd-Franklin, Hafer-Bry, & Schlecta, 2000). There is support for proactive health promotion and problem prevention as well as targeted intervention and treatment at these early ages by the use of systemic approaches that support the whole family's functioning. The Perry Preschool Project, Project 12-Ways, and the Yale Child Welfare Research Project, all of which are discussed by Boyd-Franklin et al. (2000), are examples of the same. The young child, a newcomer to the caregiving dyads, triads, and families, is invariably nested in a social context that is larger than the caregiving one. The socioemotional climate in family systems impacts the well-being and growth of the infant and young child. Forms and structures of families vary considerably in society today, as does the stability of the family unit and the values that are expressed in child rearing and family relationships. Therefore, it is important to be sensitized to questions of how family members view their own family situations, how they believe they are seen by others and by society, and how they compare their actual situations to perceived cultural ideals (Walsh, 1998). However, researchers continue to identify commitment in relationships as a most important source of human happiness (Walsh, 1998). Furthermore, processes of family functioning (caring, dedication, and self-sacrifice) and the experienced quality of relationships continue to be held up as resiliency factors in family life across diverse family forms (Walsh, 1998). Emerging empirical research in the field of family resiliency points to family cohesion, belief systems, and coping strategies as important factors at the level of the family unit and to parental nurturance, consistent discipline, and appropriate provision of autonomy at the level of the parenting unit (Kalil, 2003).

References

Aponte, H. J. (1994). How personal can training get? *Journal of Marital & Family Therapy, 20*(1), 3–15.

Aurobindo, S. (1972). *Letters on Yoga* (Vols. 22, 23, and 24). Pondicherry, India: Sri Aurobindo Ashram Trust.

Banerjee, L. (2000). Through a child's eyes: What's in a name and otherthoughts on social categorization in America. *The Community Psychologist, 33*(2), 16–18.

Banerjee, L., & Roy, S. (1987). Does the theory of logical types inform a theory of communications? *Journal of Genetic Psychology, 148*(4), 519–526.

Banerjee, L., & Sawyers, J. (1986). The double-bind: An empirical study of responses to inconsistent communications. *Journal of Marital & Family Therapy, 12*(4), 395–402.

Banerjee, L., & Sawyers, J. (1990). Interpreting subtle inconsistency and consistency: A developmental–clinical perspective. *Journal of Genetic Psychology, 151*(4), 515–521.

Banerjee, L., & Willingham, M. (1998). Self-awareness development. *Journal of Research and Applications in Clinical Psychology, 1*(2), 1–15.

Bateson, G. (1972). *Steps to an ecology of mind: A revolutionary approach to man's understanding of himself.* New York: Ballantine Books.

Bernstein, V. J., Hans, S. L., & Percansky, C. (1991). Advocating for the young child in need through strengthening the parent–child relationship. *Journal of Clinical Child Psychology, 20*(1), 28–41.

Bowen, M. (1985). *Family therapy in clinical practice.* Northvale, NJ: Jason Aronson.

Boyd-Franklin, N., Hafer-Bry, B., & Slechta, C. A. (2000). Research evidence for home-based, school, and community interventions. In N. Boyd-Franklin & B. Hafer-Bry (Eds.), *Reaching out in family therapy: Home-based, school, and community interventions* (pp. 181–201). New York: Guilford Press.

Capra, F. (1988). *Uncommon wisdom: Conversations with remarkable people.* New York: Bantam Books.

Carlson, V. J., & Harwood, R. L. (2000). Understanding and negotiating cultural differences concerning early developmental competence. *Zero to Three, 20*, 19–24.

Carter, B., & McGoldrick, M. (2005). *The expanded family life cycle: Individual, family, and social perspectives.* Menlo Park, NJ: Addison-Wesley.

Chien, W. W., & Banerjee, L. (2002). Caught between cultures: The young Asian American in therapy. In E. Davis-Russell (Ed.), *Handbook of multicultural education, research, intervention, and training* (pp. 210–220). San Francisco: Jossey-Bass.

Cohen, N. J., Lojkasek, M., Muir, R., & Parker, C. J. (2002). Six-month follow-up of two mother–infant psychotherapies: Convergence of therapeutic outcomes. *Infant Mental Health Journal, 23*, 361–380.

Dozier, M., Higley, E., Albus, K. E., & Nutter, A. (2002). Intervening with foster infants' caregivers: Targeting three critical needs. *Infant Mental Health Journal, 23*(5), 541–554.

Erikson, E. (1963). *Childhood and society.* New York: W. W. Norton.

Erickson, M. F. (1999). *Seeing is believing: Videotaping families and using self-observation to build on parenting strengths.* Minneapolis: Irving B. Harris Training Center for Infant and Toddler Development, University of Minnesota.

Greenspan, S. I., & Benderly, B. L. (1997). *The growth of the mind and the endangered origins of intelligence.* Reading, MA: Addison-Wesley.

Haley, J. (1973). *The psychiatric techniques of Milton H. Erickson, M.D.* New York: W. W. Norton & Co.

Haley, J. (1987). *Problem-solving therapy.* San Francisco: Jossey-Bass.

Haley, J., & Richeport-Haley, M. (2003). The art of strategic therapy. New York: Brunner/Routledge.

Hardy, R. V., & Lazloffy, T. A. (1995). The cultural genogram: Key to training culturally competent family therapists. *Journal of Marital & FamilyTherapy, 21*, 227–237.

Johnson, P., & Waldo, M. (1998). Integrating Minuchin's boundary continuum and Bowen's differentiation scale: A curvilinear representation. *Journal of Contemporary Family Therapy, 20*, 403–413.

Kalil, A. (2003). Family resilience and good child outcomes: A review of the literature. Retrieved on December 18, 2006 from www.msd.govt.nz/documents/publications/csre/family resilience-good-child-outcomes.pdf

Kerr, M. E., & Bowen, M. (1988). *Family evaluation: The role of the family as an emotional unit that governs individual behavior and development.* New York: W. W. Norton.

Lieberman, A. F., Silverman, J. H., & Pawl, J. H. (2000). Infant–parent psychotherapy: Core concepts and recent developments. In C. H. Zeanah (Ed.), *Handbook of infant mental health* (2nd ed., pp. 472–484). New York: Guilford Press.

McGoldrick, M., Gerson, R., & Shellenberger, S. (1999). *Genograms: Assessment and intervention.* New York: Guilford Press.

Minuchin, P., Colapinto, J., & Minuchin, S. (1998). *Working with families of the poor.* New York: Guilford Press.

Minuchin, S. (1974). *Families and family therapy.* Cambridge, MA: Harvard University Press.

Minuchin, S., Montalvo, B., Guerney, Jr., B. G., Rosman, B. L., & Schumer, F. (1967). *Families of the slums.* New York: Basic Books.

Minuchin, S., & Nichols, M. (1993). *Family healing: Strategies for hope and understanding.* New York: Simon & Schuster.

Palazolli, M. S., Boscolo, L., Cecchin, G., & Prata, G. (1978). *Paradox and counterparadox. A new model in the therapy of the family in schizophrenic transaction* (E. V. Burt, Trans.). New York: Jason Aronson. (Original work published 1975)

Rothbaum, F., & Morelli, G. (2005). Attachment and culture: Reciprocal contributions of cross-cultural research and developmental psychology. In W. Friedlmeier, P. Chakkarath, & B. Schwarz (Eds.), *Culture and human development: The importance of cross-cultural research for the social sciences* (pp. 99–123). New York: Psychology Press.

Siegal, D. J. (1999). *The developing mind.* New York: Guilford Press.

Skowron, E. A., & Schmidtt, T. A. (2003). Assessing interpersonal fusion: Reliability and validity of a new DSI Fusion With Others subscale. *Journal of Marital & Family Therapy, 29,* 209–222.

Titelman, P. (1998). Clinical applications of Bowen family systems theory. Binghamton, NY: Haworth Press.

Walsh, F. (1998). *Strengthening family resilience.* New York: Guilford Press.

Watzlawick, P., Weakland, J., & Fisch, R. (1974). *Change: Principles of problem formation and problem resolution.* New York: W. W. Norton.

Wieder, S., & Greenspan, S. I. (2005). Developmental pathways to mental health: The DIR model for comprehensive approaches to assessment and intervention. In K. M. Finello (Ed.), *The handbook of training and practice in infant and preschool mental health* (pp. 377–401). San Francisco: Jossey-Bass.

CHAPTER 3

Self-Awareness, Presence, and the Growth of Presence

Leena Banerjee Brown

Circle Five: Self-Awareness: Clinician's Reflective Narratives

The first feeling was hunger for reality and sincerity, a desire for simplicity . . . . I want real things—music that makes holes in the sky.
—Georgia O'Keefe

It is in gaining our own freedom that we can help others gain theirs. It is in experiencing love of ourselves that we are empowered to help others love themselves.

What does self-awareness offer the multicultural infant mental health clinician? It offers two important gifts. First, it offers access and connection to subjective experiences through introspection and reflection on infancy, early childhood, and early relationships for personal and professional purposes. This information becomes available for systematic integration with early childhood knowledge obtained from observation, study, and practice. Integration of these two information sources enriches clinician awareness and deepens emotional capacity for connection and empathy through experiencing a deeper connection to oneself. It also enhances preparation for multicultural infant–family mental health work through clarifying motivations in professional work. Awareness and connectedness to self facilitate similar states toward others. These states are experiential and neural phenomena, the latter based on the fact that where attention is directed, neural firing happens, thus creating and strengthening synaptic connections (Siegal, 2006).

Second, self-awareness can open up pathways for working with ease, clarity, and flexibility in professional and clinical relationships, particularly when faced with the complexity of a network of family relationships or any complex network of relationships, such as those in organizations. How so? The self of the professional is in the room and is part of the equation in professional encounters. Lack of awareness of its effects leads it to operate invisibly, thus causing distortions in these relationships (P. Minuchin, Colapinto, & Minuchin, 1998). Awareness of self provides important information on comfort zones, areas of reactivity, areas of felt connection, energy, and passion, and how these elements come into play in a variety of contexts and relationships. Refined and growing self-awareness gives the clinician access and connection to different aspects of themselves that they can use to connect with different family members (S. Minuchin, Lee, & Simon, 1996). This facilitates the widest, most versatile use of self in professional work (S. Minuchin & Fishman, 1981). Awareness and facility, with this fuller data set that consists of what the client brings in and what the professional brings in, enables professionals to become in touch with both on a moment-to-moment basis in the professional encounter, to differentiate one from the other, and to consciously use this information in their work (Banerjee & Willingham, 1998).

Empathy for infants and young children frequently comes easier for clinicians than does empathy for caregivers and other adults in the family, especially when these caregivers are unattuned or misattuning with the young child. In other words, the traps of a polarized connection with the child can make a clinician a child advocate rather than a relationship advocate. Self-awareness development processes can be very helpful in bringing to light the specific types of unattuned dynamics; the particular types of personalities, words, intonations, and interactions that can get the clinician off track in the process of connecting with family members; and the reasons in the clinician's personal story in which these obstructions are embedded. The clinician then has freedom and flexibility in negotiating the clinical process constructively. This awareness garnering is a process; it has its own rhythm and timing. Clinicians seize upon new awareness and make new choices when they are ready. Attuned collegial support and guidance in reflective supervision contexts can function synchronously with what a clinician needs as well as with what her colleagues in the group need for professional development and learning. The experience of learning in such a collegial process helps clinicians gain personal authority, professional maturity (Boszormenyi-Nagy & Krasner, 1986; Williamson, 1981), and facility in empathizing with different aspects of a relationship and with all members of a family. The ability to support whole relationships provides direct support for the natural relationship systems in a young child's life, building its inherent strengths and responding to its needs.

In 1991, the American Psychological Association's (APA) National Council for Schools of Professional Psychology (NCSPP) created a valuable document called the *Core Curriculum in Professional Psychology*. It delineated the key competencies in the training of professional psychologists, describing the relationship competency as a foundational competency (Polite & Bourg, 1991). Professional training in self-awareness development belongs in the domain of this competency. It involves training in relationships through increasing knowledge of the self and of interpersonal relationships. This learning is achieved through reflection and collegial support that catalyzes professional growth and directly teaches about catalyzing desired growth and change in clients. It is more than a purely cognitive or purely emotion-focused approach. It is an integrative one in which the visceral, emotional, and cognitive elements are brought into awareness and are integrated. Cultural context and cultural values affecting the process (Aponte, 1985) are brought to awareness and are integrated, as well. This process has been thought to be valuable in motivating and unleashing professional development (Kerr, 1981). Clinicians may enter this training process with trepidation or enthusiasm, but they find it to be of great value to their development, in my teaching and supervising experience, and in those of others (Keiley et al., 2002).

Reflective practice has been embraced in multicultural infant–family mental health, especially in supervision (Fenichel, 1992) and leadership (Parlakian & Seibel, 2001). Personal therapy has long been a requirement in analytic training and in clinical psychology training. Self-awareness development training bears resemblance to therapy but is not therapy in that the focus is specific to personal factors that relate to professional issues for which the clinician actively takes responsibility and which the clinician addresses for purposes of professional development. This focus on the self of the professional is aimed at supportively opening professionals up to themselves through encouraging and modeling vulnerability, discipline, and freedom (Aponte, 1994). This kind of training

> *allows a trainee . . . to feel all the personal emotions operating in her in a therapy session because trainers and the group take care of her while watching out for her clients. It opens up the door between the personal and the professional while strengthening boundaries. It helps achieve permeability while maintaining clarity. . . . It helps achieve integration with differentiation* (Aponte, 1994, p. 14).

The approach and strategies offered here are in sync with existing reflective approaches in multicultural infant–family mental health. They also bring new tools to the field from clinical psychology, family therapy, and multicultural psychology.

Self-awareness development practices have been systematically incorporated into family systems training for several decades, propelled by the need to prepare trainees to face the immediate and great process challenges posed by having several clients in the room at the same time. These approaches use different routes to the same ends, with some based in Bowenian work (Banerjee, 2000a; Banerjee & Willingham, 1998; Bowen, 1985; J. M. B. Keller & Protinsky, 1984); some in structural work (Aponte, 1992, 1994; Aponte & Winter, 1987); some in family sculpting work (Kane, 1996; Satir, 1987), and still others in narrative work (Lowe, 2000). These approaches increase the clinician's awareness of their own needs, of how their history and values interact with their clinical approaches and experiences of work, their needs for self-care, and their native strengths and resources. This helps a similar sensibility, curiosity, and respect to arise in attitudes toward clients and increases the acuity of the clinician's sense and understanding of a client's individuality in context.

At Alliant International University's California School of Professional Psychology at Los Angeles, at which doctoral-level clinical psychology training is provided with an active focus on multicultural psychology and serving of the underserved, self-awareness development is supported through conventions and knowledge bases in family systems therapy, multicultural psychology, and clinical psychology. It is incorporated into the doctoral training program in several ways—class discussion, written papers, field assignments, and instructor modeling in a variety of classes, especially in advanced classes. In addition, it is the focus of some process-oriented advanced clinical courses such as one that I teach in which I use an updated Bowenian model. Further modification of this model has led to its application in an ongoing training process at Early Connections, a multicultural infant–family community mental health program. Information about these modifications and experiences follows.

In 1984, J. M. B. Keller and Protinsky created a model to guide self-awareness development in family therapy trainees. This model has the following components: investigation of differentiation through genograms (Bowen, 1985) of early childhood recollections; current and recurrent dreams (as formulated by Adler (Ansbacher & Ansbacher, 1956); and sibling constellation influences (Toman, 1993). The model is in line with Bowenian practices of going home and adds to it the additional elements of early childhood recollections and dreams, thus intensifying the differentiation process so that more can be accomplished in less time (J. M. B. Keller & Protinsky, 1984). Reflections on these strands of data are brought together and shared in collegial groups that meet regularly. Countertransference issues are reflectively identified, and collegial support and insights are brought to bear on strategies for managing these issues. Ethnic identity development, one's relationship with diversity, and resiliency (Banerjee, 2000a; Banerjee & Willingham, 1998) are reflectively and collaboratively discussed.

The experience of using this self-awareness development model in the training of multicultural infant mental health clinicians at Early Connections has taught the following. The group needs a leader with experience, competence, and passion for self-awareness development processes. The leader follows and leads, facilitates, and holds and guides the process with empathy, compassion, and professional expertise. The leader must be well-versed and well-grounded in legal and ethical issues relevant to training and to the dual qualities (not dual relationships) and complexities of this particular type training (Aponte, 1994; Banerjee & Willingham, 1998). The leader also must be self-aware and committed to ongoing self-awareness development about her supervision style, strengths, needs, and resources so that she can remain genuinely engaged, effective, balanced, and able to flow with the developmental progress of the group. This self-awareness enables her to supervise competently as well as serve as an active role model who handles the personal–professional border with integrity. The process needs a programmatic and institutional culture that understands, supports, and values in-depth, reflective, collaborative approaches to training and development. This work is a first step in an ongoing journey and is supported by three principles: commitment to care for self, commitment to care for contexts in which the self functions, and commitment to deepening awareness and presence in one's life and professional work.

Small groups of no more than six to eight members are suitable for self-awareness development reflective groups. Perry's (2003) suggestion that our brains are wired so that we can connect in-depth in groups of close to six members is a useful idea to keep in mind. Ground rules should be established at the outset (Banerjee & Willingham, 1998), most especially two rules: (a) that entry into the process is a considered and volitional individual decision and (b) that confidentiality of process and content is maintained at all times, not for legal reasons but for ethical ones as a mark of professionalism and for the purpose of securing the trust necessary for the work of the group. Safety and trust are essential in the group for growth to occur and to be sustained. It is also of great value to experience trust in a training context, as it is the most essential ingredient in effective clinical relationships in multicultural infant–family mental health, as in clinical relationships in general.

In Early Connections, relevant readings were organized and shared by the leader. These readings included the journal articles on the Bowen-based training model that was used; these journal articles contained illustrations on locating natural strengths and resiliencies and building resilience by shifting from places of countertransference to places of flexibility. Supplementary readings included Ansbacher and Ansbacher (1956), Bowen (1985), Sulloway (1996), and Toman (1993) as well as examples of early childhood recollections such as Hellen Keller's (1903/2002) graphic accounts of her early sensations, emotions, and thoughts in *The Story of My Life*. Readings on ethnic identity development processes (Banerjee, 2000b, 2004; Rastogi & Wieling, 2004; Yi & Shorter-Gooden, 1999) were shared, and group members were encouraged to bring reading materials that were informative and expressive of their histories. The presentation process was initiated and modeled by the leader, a key step in building trust and leveling the playing field so that a collaborative process could unfold. Group members then took turns sharing their reflections, and the group engaged in a peer journeying facilitated by the leader.

This collaborative leadership is crucial in many ways. It ensures a climate of awareness, openness, support, and respect for the diversity of experiences shared. It is attentive to the role of culture and to the dynamics of oppression and exclusion in everyday social interactions and ordinary institutional life without replaying it through some form of hierarchy (e.g., group members do the exercises, but the leader does not). This collaborative leadership emphasizes the healing, empowering experiences of new insights, genuine peer support, and relationships in the professional development journey. In Early Connections, evaluations following the leader's modeling of her reflections generated the following types of feedback:

The modeling that was provided was particularly significant. Your openness and reflection gives us permission to do the same. The genogram presentation, in particular, engaged me on a very deep level. The vulnerability you showed makes it easier to be vulnerable.

The explicit message about the incredible personal and professional value of self-awareness (was significant). The experiential component was the most valuable aspect and could stand on its own. . . . So far, I had been very much invested in seeing myself as an individual and can now see how my struggles are shared by others in my context. In place of isolation, this awareness connects me to them.

[M]aking the connection between family history and infant development is essential. . . . I enjoyed the readings. I believe they brought meaning to the discussions. I would have to say that the readings on Helen Keller were the most helpful.

The deep-rooted connections to past family history and the dynamics that develop (were most significant) . . . I would like to look at this more in a personal/professional capacity.

The genogram presentation was amazing. The clarity of the presentation was especially helpful in formulating my own thoughts regarding my own genogram work.

The first step is development of a three- to four-generation (or more) genogram of one's own family, including in it sibling constellation issues. This step can, in itself, be a powerful process leading to new connections with old experiences that interweave understandings of relationships in early childhood, family, and culture. For example, for me, the warming of mustard oil with a few onion seeds followed by a vigorous whole-body massage by my mother or nanny was a regular feature of life in my early years. There was also the experience of one of my grandmothers taking the cream off the top of a freshly boiled pot of milk and massaging it all over my face on summer mornings when we visited her. With the buttery, creamy smell all over me, I would then bathe, and afterward, my skin would glow and I would carry with me a general sense of well-being. These smells, sounds, visual images, physical sensations, feelings, and actions from routine early experiences bring back good feelings and new awareness of familial familial–cultural rhythms of life. Reflections on differentiated patterns, as in the previous examples, can be contrasted with patterns of fusion/disengagement/triangulation and sibling constellation factors as they impact personality functioning described in the research (Sulloway, 1996; Toman,1993). These steps were taken in Early Connections, and personal experiences of strengths and vulnerabilities were articulated in lived cultural contexts and in intergenerational family histories. Group discussion followed and covered the nuances of these patterns. Peers commented on the way they heard and experienced these patterns, the way the presenter carried and presented the information, and the implications for resilience and countertransference in multicultural infant–family mental health practice. New ideas, information, and strategies were shared that applied to expanding resilient aspects and strengthening vulnerable ones. The collaborative and meaningful nature of the journey in the company of peers built deeper linkages to one's personal history, resources, and connections to one's professional work. These linkages became a source of vitalizing energy, confidence, and new knowledge.

After group members completed their genograms, presentations, and discussions, another round was held on *early childhood recollections* (ERs) as formulated by Adler (Ansbacher & Ansbacher, 1956). These ERs rely on episodic memory that contains a sense of the self (Siegal, 2006). Exploration of these memories bring rich opportunities to revisit and rediscover early familial–cultural events and the textures, sound, touch, and smells that they carry. Similar supportive and reflective peer journeying occurred on the feelings, meanings, drives, and motivations inherent in chosen and remembered ERs. Discussion focused on how these feelings, meanings, drives, and motivations speak to multicultural infant–family mental health work and enrich it; and where there are barriers to relationship and empathy.

Early ethnic or sociocultural identity was discussed in terms of early messages received from caregivers, family members, day care/preschool personnel, and community members. The effects of those messages in terms of positive self-feelings; sense of agency; and feelings of discrimination, exclusion, invisibility, and internalized racism were reflected on, voiced, seen, and heard. The group leader encouraged reflections on stories, mythology, customs, celebrations, heroines and heroes, artwork, music, and the rhythms of daily life (Banerjee, 2002) in this early environment. One innovation that was introduced and enthusiastically received by the group was the choice of sharing early photographs during this process. These photographs afforded rich opportunities for new observations and connections with family culture as well as early states of regulation and dyadic attunement. It was very interesting for me, for example, to hear group members point out my apparent collected inward state in my paternal grandfather's arms at age 1, contrasted with a photograph taken on the very same time and day in which I appeared collected and gregarious in my paternal grandmother's arms. It led me to notice and reflect on the distinctly different personalities of the two adults, and their different physical (and relational/dyadic) ways of holding of me in the photographs.

Another round followed in which current and any recurrent dreams were looked at from an Adlerian perspective. The group pondered information on those personal goals that positively affect personal and professional relationships and that benefit the community (goals that Adler describes as being on the side of social interest) and those personal goals that obstruct such relationships (goals that Adler describes as being on the socially useless side). Strengths were recognized and strategies were considered where struggles were acknowledged. Consider the following example of a particular theme explored through these three consecutive presentations:

As the initiator of the Early Connections self-awareness development reflective process, I began with my early experiences with loss. My four-generation genogram connected me to numerous, recurrent experiences of loss through illness and premature death in at least two prior generations of my father's family. There were instances of unexpected and premature loss in my mother's family, too, but this loss was less pervasive. For my mother, though, there was loss of freedom, choice, and developmental opportunity through early marriage arranged by her patriarchical family. For my father, too, there was early loss of freedom, choice, and opportunity resulting from taking a route to early employment. As an only son of an ailing father, he felt it to be his unspoken duty to stand on his own feet and be a man, a less often considered side of the pressures of patriarchy. These family experiences occurred in the context of a society that was still emerging from the devastating psychological realities of colonization involving the loss of liberty, dignity, agency, and economic resources. The impact of two centuries of foreign domination and oppression left its mark on people in the society in many ways including the bias toward "fair skin and sharp features" that many in the family and, indeed, the society did not have. However in a civilization as old (at least 5,000 years) and as complex as India, it is hard to accurately trace the roots of such internalized racism, as these have had many different opportunities to set in and take root. For me, a girl child who was neither fair skinned nor sharp featured, there was loss of an inarticulable form in the absence of communal celebration of my physical being, a feeling that doubtless was shared by many others who were like me. Such can be the unspeakable, tragic nature and reverberations of oppression in its collectively internalized aspects.

In my family (a large, interconnected, extended family), there was unwavering love, complex and stable networks of family relationships, education, erudition, varied social achievements, many stellar accomplishments, beauty, generosity, integrity, capacity for sacrifice, loyalty, and dedication. These elements remained alive amidst the harshness of the losses and trials and the fragilities and roadblocks caused by the emotionally unresolved status of some of them.

As a firstborn infant and young girl child in this family emotional and cultural context, I had much privilege as well as much (too much) expectation upon me. The special qualities of each of my parents' attunement to me were part of a context of other attunements of grandparents, nannies, aunts and uncles, and cousins as well as my parents' colleagues and close friends. I was born slightly premature after an extended labor but flourished in every respect except for the slow appearance of hair on my head and teeth in my mouth! I had an easy temperament and a sociable nature, and my first birthday photographs depict me in bald, cherubic form cutting a big chocolate cake in the form of a ship held by my mother surrounded by older peers. My linguistic environment was rich with at least three (and sometimes more) languages spoken routinely. Ease and facility of multilingualism and openness to linguistic diversity was amply modeled by members of my family. As a toddler, I spoke early and became multilingual in a natural way. I was impatient about being let into the neighborhood preschool and used my toddler vocabulary to badger my family about it, eventually succeeding in entering one long before my time.

My younger siblings were born in quick succession, when I was 2 and 4, increasing the demands on my parents' time and energy and limiting their emotional availability to me. My paternal grandfather was very ill in my infancy and passed away by the time I was 2. My young father felt this to be the deepest loss of his life. When I was still a very young child, my father was deployed at the Indo-Chinese border to fight in a war, an event that occurred twice more in my childhood, taking him then to the Indo-Pak border. I compensated with these stresses in the family environment with parentified responses, leading me to be the good, obedient child and elder sister, although I was only a close peer to my siblings. I gave no trouble and was no trouble, and in this process, I lost my own voice. I had very regular bouts of tonsillitis instead, times when my mother treated me with a kind of attuned care and attention that I sorely needed.

My reflections have helped me to connect with difficult early feelings, fear, anger, and guilt that I felt and had suppressed, as I had felt no room to voice them then. These were legitimate needs at my age—to be carefree and understood rather than be understanding. I was particularly sensitive to my mother's fears and anxieties for my father's safety and well-being when my father was away and at war, and I absorbed some of her fears. I was also sensitive to her frustrations and anger at various members in the family network with whom, at the time, she could not effectively negotiate her relationships and be heard. Because we lived with my paternal grandmother in our ancestral home at the time, I was sensitive to my grandmother's grief as well in the years following my paternal grandfather's death. I was aware of the discomfort of such feelings as they circulated about in the family context, although I could neither identify nor articulate them then. I did not act them out, either; I suppressed them, something that an easy-tempered, eldest girl child in a relatively patriarchical family and society may be apt to do.

It is no great surprise that one of my earlier memories is about my newborn youngest sister coming home from the hospital with my mother to our ancestral home. I was 4 years old. It is likely that the arrival of my middle sister when I was 2 was even more significant to the changes I experienced in my circumstances. But this I do not have in explicit memory, possibly for developmental reasons and possibly for emotional ones. In the ERs I have feelings of nurturance toward my new sibling and relief in the return of my mother, more readily than feelings of discomfort with the new situation. There may have been anxiety, fear or anger in the situation for me because it had happened before, and because there may have been unattended-to loss involved in it for me.

Reflections have helped me reconnect with these times in my life, to own the pleasures and the displeasures in them, and to accept both in my story. These experiences have been freeing and have taken me to a more easy, flexible, and neutral place for working with challenging emotions in relationships with clients. These experiences have contributed to my ability to hold difficult issues, tolerate the intensities and ambiguities that arise in processing them, and be patient in letting resolution occur organically and in a way that empowers clients. In time this has evolved into a style of facilitating reflective supervision in a similar way, a style that has worked well for supervisees and has felt in sync with me.

The strong capacity for empathy that I experienced almost osmotically in early relationships and family environments is something that I recognized to be a critical strength for me in my work as a healer (psychologist), teacher (professor, clinical supervisor), and author, for my style is based on connectedness. Returning to the early roots of my experiences with empathy strengthens my clarity about what belongs to me, what belongs in another, and what flows back and forth in the relationship. It gives me new appreciation of my own empathic abilities and renewed courage to face both strengths and vulnerabilities in self and in relationships. Such reflections provide a disciplined path to freedom from emotional caretaking and realization of the full potential of my innate and developed capacity for empathy.

From this journey I know again that the early environment contains powerful and important messages about self including race, ethnicity, gender, ability, and class that give the infant and young child an inchoate but growing sense of who they are in sociocultural context. Similarly, there are sights, smells, textures, and tastes of foods and people, sounds and movements of lullabies, and songs and dances that tell them about who they are in this context. I know from reconnecting with such messages how important they are to making sense of oneself at the roots of the identity development process. Adults around infants and young children may or may not be aware of the significance of these early sensory–affective–cognitive messages for them, but they are invested in passing on their cultural roots to them. These are important opportunities for shaping an early sense of comfort and well-being in one's skin and in the skin of one's family and community. Such comfort sets the foundations for healthy ethnic identity development and sense of belonging in a familial–sociocultural context. I know that awareness raising and attunement refining is an infinite journey, as well, in which we can all only commit to being lifelong students.

My current dreams have frequently centered on this theme of claiming voice, of routes to finding authentic voice and contexts that authentically resonate with it. Writing this book is a big part of claiming my voice for myself but also for my family, teachers, peers, and students, all those individuals on whose shoulders I stand and all those who hold my hands. Most of all, I write for unborn, newborn, and young children, the hope of our species. I write also for my children, their children, the children I know and those with whom I have worked so that they may thrive and we may help them.

This is the self-awareness development model used at Early Connections. If implemented weekly, the process takes 6–8 weeks for each cycle/module, depending on the size of the group. The group can then create variations and elaborations in collaborative consultation with one another on the basis of their assessment of their interests and needs. In Early Connections, the group has completed four steps:

1. Genograms in sociocultural context with sibling constellation influences;
2. Early childhood recollections and early sociocultural identity;
3. Current and recurrent dreams; and
4. Self-care practices (which are presented in the Circle Seven discussion).

Currently the Early Connections team is collectively discussing its choice of next steps in the self-awareness development process.

Circle Six: Clinician Presence in the Holding of Relationships (Interpersonal World)

Babies by their very existence call us back to something we all sense we have lost. They do not enchant us simply because they are "cute" but because they awaken in us a thirst that sleeps deep within some wellspring of yearning that we know we have neglected. Babies are meant to challenge some of our ideas of "normal" and to teach us not to be so blasé about our adult experience. After all, why are babies born?
—William S. Schafer, 2004 (p. 8)

If self-awareness development is about going back to one's infancy and childhood to build capacity and better prepare oneself to work in multicultural infant–family mental health, presence is about being there—in the work and in the moment—in a full and sustained way. This full presence involves the integration of the information from all previous circles. Thus the professional's presence embodies this integration, and objectively and subjectively informed awareness flows through this presence into relationships. How much of ourselves is present and in the room with the infant, the young child, their parent(s), and family? If we measured this on a scale of 1 to 10, how much of us is here today and how much of us will be here in a sampling of sessions over a period of time? Aggregating this information, what is our range of presence in our clinical role in multicultural infant–family mental health? What is the quality of this presence? Is there enjoyment in it? Is there the ability to hold a range of feelings and events? What are the barriers to presence? All of us feel some version of lighting up, that demeanor of joy in Berry Brazelton that still blows me away when he comes into the presence of a newborn. I feel that lighting up, too, and I see it and hear about it in my peers. These feelings tell me that this work in multicultural infant–family mental health is ours to do.

How do we capture this positive experience in a working definition of presence? Bugental (1978), writing in humanistic psychology, defined *presence* as genuine and complete absorption in activity and intent to participate to full capacity, remain accessible to others, and be expressive of self. The two elements of absorption and intent to participate fully are echoed in Csikszentmihalyi's (1990) definition of *flow*. He says that flow is engagement and attentiveness with enjoyment and vitality that comes from being deeply in sync with where you are at a given time. Taking from these definitions and adding a few more from my own observations and experiences, we have the following elements, all of which give us a working definition of presence:

- Complete absorption or attentiveness. This element is reminiscent of Siegal's (1999) description of being present and lost.
- Intent to participate fully or engage.
- Accessibility/connectedness/openness to self and to expressing self.
- Accessibility/connectedness/openness to others.
- Experience of enjoyment and vitality.
- Experience of being in sync.
- Experience of aliveness, information-rich awareness, carrying a sense of well-being.

Thus, in the Circles framework, *presence* is that feeling of aliveness and connection with an infant and her family in which the clinician is fully absorbed and engaged and feels access to her own experiences and those of her clients with enjoyment, vitality, and informed awareness, being centered and in sync in the moment.

Schafer (2004) gives us a valuable developmental perspective on presence. In an infant, he describes presence as "pure awareness—void of content, free from all internal commentary, judgment, comparison, fear, or desire" (p. 5). This is the state in a quiet, alert infant, a state that, Schafer observes, makes joy and awareness of other's awareness possible. He describes joy as being open and drawn toward "something or someone in wonder, curiosity, and interest, without any fear or impulse to reject" (p. 5). Schafer reminds us that the capacity to experience such joy, to hold it and abide with it, is a capacity that infants are born with and, therefore, one that we all have. Awareness of others' awareness, Schafer notes, is a capacity that becomes apparent some months after birth and within the first year of life. It is, he observes, the capacity for shared attention and communication. Perhaps it is also the capacity for early connectedness to self and others, the rudiments of empathy—a capacity that we come hard wired for and one that neuroscience is actively demonstrating to be so.

Thus, a newborn infant has the experience of presence in terms of his experience of being in the moment leading to experiences of joy as well as connectedness to self (savoring own experiences) and to others. Becoming aware of one's presence is something that comes later with the capacity for reflection. Being able to work with one's presence is a capacity that comes with adult reflective practices such as the reflective self-awareness development exercises discussed in the earlier section. Thus, these three progressive aspects of presence—the experience of presence; the awareness of one's presence; and the capacity to work with it, enhance it, and expand it—are developmental in nature. Presence is an important process with which multicultural infant–family mental health clinicians can engage as it lies at the core of infant–family experience and facilitates engagement with the rich silences, preverbal utterances, and nonverbal communications between infants/young children and their parents, caregivers, family members, and clinicians.

Schafer (2004) makes a unique and eloquent call for collaborating and learning from infants about those fundamentally integrative aspects of development and ultimate developmental tasks with which we have lost connection and, therefore, have no way to teach our children. The reason for our loss, he states, is the inability to integrate the spiritual dimension of development into our knowledge base of human development. This lack of integration results in a knowing silence about it. Such is the case with every fundamental aspect of reality that pushes the envelope of our comfort zones. Multicultural psychology that has lead the reexamination of mental illness and well-being in sociocultural/political/historical context has been confronting aspects of this same silence. This is a silence about the wholeness of reality and, in the case of multicultural psychology, about current, ongoing, and sometimes muted forms of oppression that continue in our worlds and in each of our experiences. The refusal to acknowledge parts of reality that do not fit mental conceptions of who we are—and the refusal to admit and explore spirit, soul, and synchronicity that we can all experience because they may challenge the limitations of the traditional, faltering, scientific paradigm—leaves us with a fractured worldview, information base, and strategies for action. This distorts what we know and what we do with it, especially when it comes to knowledge about the human species, for whom connection, identity, meaning, awareness, joy, development, and belonging are of paramount significance. Any endeavor to integrate and reclaim wholeness in paradigms of knowledge and follow it through to societal and institutional shifts in mindset, culture, policy, and practice is an endeavor to develop and transform our collective state of awareness and existence. This kind of progress can be measured directly in individual, relational, and collective states of presence.

Thich Nat Hanh, the renowned author and Vietnamese Buddhist monk, led a peace walk at MacArthur Park in Los Angeles in 2005. In this beautiful park, in a crime-ridden, urban community of poor, immigrant children and families, he spoke about practices that support our abilities to be present, to be in the here and now. He spoke of how to walk, sit, and eat meditatively and mindfully, offering simple guidance for profound shifts in awareness, intention, experience, and action. I took this walk with Thich Nat Hanh and many hundred fellow citizens. At one point in the walk, not knowing quite how I got there, I found myself walking beside Thich Nat Hanh, shoulder to shoulder. In that close proximity I experienced him as an embodiment of every member of humankind. Such was the depth and focus of his calm and the even, openness, and acceptance in his presence. Meditative practices, also called mindfulness practices, have been integrated into clinical practice and studied for some time. Their positive value has been reported in research (Baer, 2003) on those suffering from major depression (Segal, Williams, & Teasdale, 2002), anxiety (Miller, Fletcher, & Kabat-Zinn, 1995), borderline personality disorder (Linehan, 1993), and chronic illness and pain (Teasdale et al., 2000). Body systems that are adversely affected by stress, such as the cardiac system, the immune system, and the endocrine system, benefit and improve in their functioning through mindfulness practice (Kabat-Zinn, 2005).

In 2005, a think tank was organized by Children's Institute, Inc. in Los Angeles to create consensus on clinical guidelines for the use of such practices with traumatized children. A concept paper summarized the literature and framed the specific discussion questions. Twelve local and national experts gathered to spend the day in dialogue addressing those questions accompanied by a small audience of observers. I was an invited member of this think tank. The group was interdisciplinary, and each group member was a practitioner of some form of meditation or mindfulness practice. The meetings started with, were interspersed with, and ended with meditation practices especially created for the occasion. In the think tank discussions, we agreed that what we meant by "meditation" or "mindfulness" was awareness, a word that leaves open the possibility that the scientific paradigm, as it evolves, can make a paradigmatic shift to include spirit, mind, and body.

Kabat-Zinn (2003) operationally defined *meditation* as "the awareness that emerges through paying attention on purpose, in the present moment, and nonjudgmentally to the unfolding of experience moment by moment" (p. 145). As a physician who has developed manualized curricula for integrating meditation into interventions for stress reduction and a researcher and author who has contributed extensively to the subject, Kabat-Zinn's summary of core meditative practices are silence; stillness; self-inquiry; embodiment; emotional sensitivity; accepting the full gamut of emotional expression held in awareness; acknowledging the universal yearning for well-being, happiness, and peace; and meeting, honoring, and mobilizing this yearning for transformation. Awareness involves poetry and science, direct and indirect experience, and subjective and objective knowledge. Thus, it is taken out of the context of any particular religious practice or faith. Most important, awareness is an invitation to the self to be present.

At the think tank, my conclusions on the mechanisms underlying such awareness were that there are two sets, regulatory and attitudinal, and that they are progressive and developmental in nature (Banerjee, 2005). The regulatory set involves the self-regulation of attention and arousal to stay present. There is anchoring in breath, or concentration on a singular external element; switching or volitionally shifting focus from distracting sensations, feelings, thoughts, and memories back to the present and point of focus; monitoring and control of cognitive processes; and inhibition of secondary elaborations. This means that awareness is nonelaborative and is focused on direct experiences. These regulatory mechanisms slow down stress physiology and increase the quiet, alert state. An infant or young child, capable of pure awareness (Schafer, 2004), experiences this slowing spontaneously in an attuned, well-scaffolded, caregiving environment. When dysregulation occurs, the infant and young child depends on the caregiver's attunement to bring him back through dyadic regulation to such states of calmness and tranquility. At the think tank, there was consensus that these first set of regulatory mechanisms of centering through focus on breath or any external object for achievement of a quiet, alert state was not contraindicated for anyone at any age.

The second set of mechanisms are attitudinal and have been described as focusing with quiet alertness on the present moment and being open to, accepting of, and curious about each moment of experience and what it brings. It can involve increasing affect tolerance of distressing affects; shifting the meanings of difficult experiences and increasing the range of emotional awareness, presence, and psychological mindedness. We agreed that this set of mechanisms necessitated a discriminating clinical use on the basis of a trusting relationship with clients and determination of their readiness, resilience, stability, and reality orientation, ruling out those clients who were in severe crisis.

Developmentally, this second set of mechanisms does not apply to infants and young children, who can have the experience of awareness without the awareness of having it or the capacity (so far as we know) to work with it. However, this second set of mechanisms remains very relevant for the caregivers, parents, and family members of infants and young children as well as the professionals who work with them. These two sets of mechanisms are, thus, progressive steps in that one comes before the other. The practice of awareness itself also is progressive in that it deepens over time (Kabat-Zinn, 2003). Awareness raising is a practice that cannot be taught or passed on as a parent/caregiver or a professional without the experience and practice of raising one's own awareness or the experience of integrating this practice with psychotherapy practice. Kabat-Zinn quotes T. S. Eliot in describing awareness as a condition of complete simplicity that is the "work of a lifetime. . . . and the work of no time at all" (p. 149). Awareness-raising practices such as reflective dialogue, self-reflection, meditation, contemplation, spiritual practice, and continuing education classes on these subjects sustain and build presence.

Circle Seven: Creating Sustaining Space: Personally–Culturally Meaningful Self-Care, Generating Presence (Simultaneous Access to Intrapersonal and Interpersonal Worlds)

If the six circles, thus far, provide a comprehensive set of parameters with which to work in multicultural infant–family mental health, then this seventh circle speaks to the contexts in which this work occurs and to relationships with that context. Context—institutional and organizational—supports the work occurring within it through its cultures, philosophies, theories, technologies, and practices. How can professionals relate to their organizations and how can these organizations support them so that they continually renew their feelings of presence and aliveness in multicultural infant–family mental health work? In answer to this question, Circles points to the roles of taking active responsibility for self–care and of creating stable, collective spaces for reflective dialogue, relationship, and collaborative organizational cultures in which presence can grow. These are the central elements that clinicians can explore in Circle Seven.

Empowerment through self-knowledge–based self-care practices that increase sense of well-being can be a place to start. Positive changes and well-being in individuals and relationships can cascade into similar changes in the environments in which they function. Ultimately, the quality of a clinician's work is related to the quality of the clinician's life in the workplace/institution and contexts beyond it. Self-care practices are, therefore, important for their potential to positively affect the clinician's ongoing experience and evolving awareness in her work. As individuals in a collective transform, their relationships transform, and the collective itself transforms; thus, self-care can be considered for its merits in helping not only clinicians but also organizations grow and transform.

At Early Connections, the multicultural infant–family mental health program mentioned in Circle Five, group members took turns making brief presentations on self-care practices that sustain their work and their lives. This presentation was a way of paying attention to these practices, bringing them into the workplace, sharing them with colleagues, enjoying collegial receptivity to them, and making room for such dialogue in the workplace. There was considerable personal–cultural variation in what was shared, as the following summary illustrates:

One of the clinicians shared her interest and work with singing bowls from observing the clinical supervisor's previous clinical work using the bowls for biobehavioral regulation with traumatized toddlers. She spoke of the way in which she paired slow, deep breathing with the practice of playing the bowl and the feelings of expansiveness that it gave her. She shared this joy with young children by playing the bowls for them and pairing them with deep breathing and visualizations relating to sensory and emotional experiences about a favorite time or place. When she did the exercise herself, she breathed deeply, visualized the sea, and played the singing bowl. It gave her space and clarity.

Another clinician spoke of connections to home and a sense of belonging, both of which center her. She shared symbolic objects such as traditional lamps and incense holders as well as ceremony and ritual involving lighting lamps, burning incense, playing ancient chants, and drawing traditional floor patterns. These practices help ground her in a meaningful and familiar cultural space that she misses in the mainstream of her everyday work life. These practices also connect her to the sacred and the timeless. This connection to her center helps keep her alive, enthusiastic, and connected in her clinical work and in her relationships.

One clinician shared how she became aware of her own capacity for bodily empathy in working with very ill children. She talked about her experience of realizing that she absorbed and held pain and stress from her young clients by tightening her body. She sought her own regulation through walking, breathing, and grounding herself through touch; creating space for herself at day's end; and sharing it in silent joy with her young son, letting the wind blow away the cares of the day as they sat together on their porch at eventide. She said that she realized that such self-care is not selfish but necessary, and the resistance to it carries both message and meaning, a deciphering that hones her nonverbal communication skills in working in multicultural infant–family mental health.

Another clinician spoke about arts and crafts activities that she enjoys, such as painting small flower pots and planting new life in them. She enjoys doing such activities with others in her family. She enjoys the variety of colors in the palate, the beauty of the painted pots, and the conversations that spontaneously arise as family members work and create together. She also uses these activities in art and play therapy with young children and their families. The choices of colors, the way of painting, the patterns drawn, and the family interactions around the activities provide good observational information for therapeutic dialogue.

Another clinician spoke of his investment in reflecting and learning from relationships in personal therapy and supervision. He shared observations of himself as being inclined toward engagement through action and, frequently, through seeking actions. At times, such insights allow him to get in touch with his early experiences and states in which these patterns may have had their genesis and increase his awareness and empathy for similar needs and dynamics of young children in families.

A clinician spoke of her weekly practice of walking up a mountain and this being a journey unto itself in which she attunes to the smells of the eucalyptus and to the sounds and sights of bees humming around her and falls into a quiet communion with herself in motion. She has observed that as time has gone on, she has begun running on this same trail. Her pace of movement has changed, and her enjoyment and commitment to the process have been deepening. She is aware that this practice rejuvenates, centers, and feeds her work through increasing her physical strength and discipline. This translates into increased power, agency, and vitality in working with young children and their caregivers.

A final clinician shared her long desire for direct experiences of the transcendent in everyday life and finding it as much through spiritual practice as through being with, seeing, and hearing young children. She spoke of her spiritual practice and of her experiences of seeing nature with and through the eyes of her very young clients, who noticed the beauty in tiny flowers blooming in the grass, details that many adults who are higher off the ground missed or took for granted. She spoke of the tenderness of the love that they could express in secure relationships by regularly giving away their newfound discoveries or treasuring those given to them by security-giving figures in their lives.

References

Ansbacher, H. L., & Ansbacher, R. R. (1956). *The individual psychology of Alfred Adler*. New York: Basic Books.

Aponte, H. J. (1985). The negotiation of values in therapy. *Family Process, 24*, 323–338.

Aponte, H. J. (1992). Training the person of the therapist in structural family therapy. *Journal of Marital & Family Therapy, 18*(3), 269–281.

Aponte, H. J. (1994). How personal can training get? *Journal of Marital & Family Therapy, 20*(1), 3–15.

Aponte, H. J., & Winter, J. E. (1987). The person and practice of the therapist: Treatment and training. *Journal of Psychotherapy and the Family, 3*, 85–111.

Baer, R. A. (2003). Mindfulness training as a clinical intervention: A conceptual and empirical review. *Clinical Psychology: Science and Practice, 10*, 125–143.

Banerjee, L. (2000a). Self-development practices for professionals: Gems from the family therapy field. *Psychological Foundations: The Journal, 11*(2), 48–54.

Banerjee, L. (2000b). Through a child's eyes: What's in a name and other thoughts on social categorization in America. *The Community Psychologist, 33*(2), 16–18.

Banerjee, L. (2002). Psychology and the reach of multiculturalism in American culture. In E. Davis-Russell (Ed.), *Handbook of multicultural education, research, intervention, and training*. San Francisco: Jossey-Bass.

Banerjee, L. (2004). Dress as a manifest aspect of identity: An Indian American narrative. In J. Chin (Ed.), *The psychology of prejudice and discrimination: Vol. 4. Disability, religion, physique and other traits* (pp. 1–26). Westport, CT: Praeger Press.

Banerjee, L. (2005). Intensive day treatment for very young traumatized children in residential care. In K. M. Finello (Ed.), *The handbook of training and practice in infant and preschool mental health* (pp. 3–30). San Francisco: Jossey-Bass.

Banerjee, L., & Willingham, M. (1998). Self-awareness development. *Journal of Research and Applications in Clinical Psychology, 1*(2), 1–15.

Boszormenyi-Nagy, I., & Krasner, B. (1986). *Between give and take: A clinical guide to contextual therapy*. New York: Brunner/Mazel.

Bowen, M. (1985). *Family therapy in clinical practice*. Northvale, NJ: Jason Aronson.

Bugental, J. F. T. (1978). *Psychotherapy and process*. Menlo Park, NJ: Addison-Wesley.

Csikszentmihalyi, M. (1990). *Flow: The psychology of optimal experience*. New York: Harper Perennial.

Fenichel, E. (Ed.). (1992). *Learning through supervision and mentorship how to support the development of infants, toddlers and their families: A source book*. Washington, DC: ZERO TO THREE.

Kabat-Zinn, J. (2003). Mindfulness-based interventions in context: Past, present and future. *Clinical Psychology: Science and Practice, 10*(2), 144–156.

Kabat-Zinn, J. (2005). *Coming to our senses: Healing ourselves and the world through mindfulness*. New York: Hyperion.

Kane, C. M. (1996). An experiential approach to marital and family therapy trainees. *Journal of Marital & Family Therapy, 22*, 481–487.

Keiley, M. K., Dolbin, M., Hill, J., Karrupaswamy, N., Liu, T., Natrajan, R., et al. (2002). The cultural genogram: Experiences from within a marriage and family therapy training program. *Journal of Marital and Family Therapy, 28*(2), 165–178.

Keller, H. (1903/2002). *The story of my life*. Repr. New York: Signet Classic.

Keller, J. M. B., & Protinsky, H. (1984). A self-management model of supervision. *Journal of Marital & Family Therapy, 10*, 281–288.

Kerr, M. E. (1981). Family systems theory and therapy. In A. S. Gurman and D. P. Kniskern (Eds.), *Handbook of Family Therapy* (pp. 226–264). New York: Brunner/Mazel.

Lowe, R. (2000). Supervising self-supervision: Constructive inquiry and embedded narratives in case consultation. *Journal of Marital & Family Therapy, 26*, 511–521.

Linehan, M. M. (1993). *Cognitive behavioral treatment of borderline personality disorders*. New York: Guilford Press.

Miller, J. J., Fletcher, K., and Kabat-Zinn, J. (1995). Three year follow up and clinical implications of a mindfulness meditation based stress reduction intervention in the treatment of anxiety disorders. *General Hospital Psychiatry, 17,* 192–200.

Minuchin, P., Colapinto, J., & Minuchin, S. (1998). *Working with families of the poor.* New York: Guilford Press.

Minuchin, S., & Fishman, C. H. (1981). *Family therapy techniques.* Cambridge, MA: Harvard University Press.

Minuchin, S., Lee, W. Y., & Simon, G. M. (1996). *Mastering family therapy.* New York: Wiley.

Parlakian, R., & Seibel, N. L. (2001). *Being in charge: Reflective leadership in infant/family programs.* Washington, DC: ZERO TO THREE.

Perry, B. (2003, May). *Nature and nurture of brain development.* Paper presented at the From Neurons to Neighborhoods Conference, Los Angeles, CA. Retrieved on December 21, 2006, from www.childtrauma.org

Polite, K., & Bourg, E. (1991). Relationship competency. In R. L. Peterson, J. D. McHolland, R. J. Bent, E. Davis-Russell, G. E. Edwall, K. Polite, et al. (Eds.), *The core curriculum in professional psychology* (pp. 83–88). Washington, DC: American Psychological Association.

Rastogi, M., & Wieling, E. (Eds.). (2004). *Voices of color: First person accounts of ethnic minority therapists* (pp. 297–312). Thousand Oaks, CA: Sage.

Satir, V. (1987). The therapist story. *Journal of Psychotherapy and the Family, 3,* 17–23.

Schafer, W. (2004). The infant as reflection of soul: The time before there was a self. *Zero to Three, 24,* 4–8.

Segal, Z. V., Williams, J. M. G., & Teasdale, J. D. (2002). *Mindfulness-based cognitive therapy for depression: A new approach to preventing relapse.* New York: Guilford Press.

Siegal, D. J. (1999). *The developing mind: Towards a neurobiology of interpersonal experience.* New York: Guilford Press.

Siegal, D. J. (2006, March). *Awakening the mind to the wisdom of the body.* Paper presented at The Embodied Mind: Integration of the Body, Brain, and Mind in Clinical Practice: A UCLA Extension and Lifespan Learning Institute Conference, Los Angeles, CA.

Sulloway, F. J. (1996). *Born to rebel: Birth order, family dynamics, and creative lives.* New York: Pantheon.

Teasdale, J. D., Segal, J. V., Williams, J. M. G., Ridgeway, V. A., Soulsby, J., & Lau, M. (2000). Prevention of relapse recurrence in major depression by mindfulness-based cognitive therapy. *Journal of Consulting and Clinical Psychology, 68,* 615–623.

Toman, W. (1993). *Family constellation: Its effects on personality and social behavior.* Northvale, NJ: Jason Aronson.

Williamson, D. (1981). Personal authority via termination of the intergenerational hierarchical boundary: A "new" stage in the family life cycle. *Journal of Marital & Family Therapy, 7,* 441–452.

Yi, K., & Shorter-Gooden, K. (1999). Ethnic identity formation: From stage theory to a constructivist narrative model. *Psychotherapy, 36,* 16–26.

PART II: CHRONICLES OF CLINICAL CASE APPLICATIONS

CHAPTER 4

Kevin's Early Infancy: Regulation and Well-Being Through Innovations in Multicultural Infant–Family Mental Health

Leena Banerjee Brown

Introduction

Kevin is a 3-month-old African American infant who was referred for multicultural infant–family mental health services with his Hispanic American foster family. He is a high-risk infant with multiple medical and psychosocial risk factors and multiple experiences of hidden and unhidden traumas. He is in frequent intense distress, is affectively fearful, cries excessively and inconsolably, and has difficulties in feeding, resting, and sleeping. He presents with posttraumatic stress disorder and regulatory disorder of hypersensitivity—Type A: Fearful/cautious in the *Diagnostic Classification of Mental Health and Developmental Disorders of Infancy and Early Childhood (DC:0–3R)* diagnostic classification system (ZERO TO THREE, 2005). This case illustrates the use of the Circles framework in engaging with Kevin in his new foster family and in building his foundations of healthy regulation, attachment, and identity. New research illuminating the infant and young child's experience of trauma and providing the basis for innovative, regulating interventions using touch and sound are summarized.

Presenting Problem

Kevin, a 3-month old African American baby, was born at 37 weeks' gestation, the cusp of prematurity (Browne, 2004) and spent the first month of life in the hospital. His next 2 months were spent in family foster care before he came to his current Hispanic American foster family. A medically fragile infant and the child of a substance-abusing mother, he was screened in the hospital for retinopathy of prematurity and was diagnosed with incomplete vascularization of both eyes. He was also followed and treated for bronchial distress and wheezing.

Kevin's eyes were bright, prominent, and expressive. You noticed them right away, as you did his full head of raven hair. He was exposed to crack cocaine in utero, and he cried excessively throughout the day and night, totaling many hours each and every day. It took a long time, at least a half hour at a time, before he was soothed. He slept and rested very little and very fitfully and, in his caregiver's words, "went up and down all night and all day." In his waking state, he was alert but restless. He did not feed well, his rooting and sucking were weak, and he vomited his food several times a day in substantial quantity. He was a thin, small, wiry, dark baby, and his incredibly taut, hypertonic limbs shook with tremors. He arched his back when he was held. His startle reflex, or Moro reflex, worked overtime; he startled numerous times every day, his facial expressions retracting in fear and apprehension as his limbs thrust out and trembled. He made eye contact and stared at people, sometimes in a hyperalert manner, but rarely, if ever, did he smile at anyone. On rare occasions when he smiled at his caregiver, he gave her a very slight, if crooked, smile. His hyperalert stare gave the impression, at times, of intense fright akin to panic. He had developed an umbilical hernia, and his congestion had progressed into bronchiolitis.

Family and Placement History

Kevin is the 23rd child of his African American mother. She has a longstanding and entrenched history of substance abuse, prostitution, poverty, and unstable residence. She has also had a longstanding relationship with child protection authorities, as 17 of her children are dependents of the court. Seven of these 17 children have been permanently placed with new families, and her parental rights with them have been terminated. Kevin's mother has tried and failed to avail of the rehabilitation services provided to her. The connection between her and service providers who have reached out to her has been tenuous and invariably broken, and she has remained beyond their reach. She came into a hospital to deliver Kevin. After giving birth, she walked away, a lone and desolate figure in extreme anguish, utter desperation, and pain. She gave Kevin his name but did not otherwise connect with him at all. She was not able to identify Kevin's father, and no man came forward to claim him.

One of Kevin's older sisters, a 19-year-old girl, stepped forward and was deemed as having adequate support and ability to provide for his care when he was discharged from the hospital. This was his first placement in kinship care. This decision soon proved to be unworkable, and in a couple of months, his sister contacted authorities for help in placing him elsewhere. His multiple medical needs and his routine care needs were overwhelming for her.

Three months after birth, Kevin was placed in a Hispanic American foster family and was referred for both multicultural infant–family mental health services and regional center services. He had experienced changes in his primary caregivers and early caregiving environment three times in his first 3 months of extrauterine life. His intrauterine life was spent in his mother's conditions of poverty, instability, transience, substance use, lack of prenatal care and social support, and undeterminable nutritional support.

Mental Health Interventions and Outcomes

A comprehensive psychosocial assessment of Kevin in his foster family—an assessment that included in-depth interviewing and multiple behavior observations during feeding and sleeping and in crying/distressed and nondistressed states—led to the establishment of a good working relationship and a treatment focus on regulation and attachment. His foster mother was following up with all of his medical appointments for treating his congestion and for monitoring his vision and umbilical hernia. She was using, as advised, a saline suction device and a nebulizer that aided his breathing and recovery from bronchiolitis. She was giving him his prescribed medications and his new hypoallergenic formula. His foster mother had extensive prior experience with caring for medically fragile infants in a group home. She had transitioned from doing that work to becoming a foster parent, and Kevin was her first foster child. Thus, Kevin came to a quiet, settled home of two older foster parents who had raised their own four children. Three of their adult children led independent lives, lived nearby, and visited often with their families. One of their children, a son, had been developmentally delayed and passed away from medical complications 1 year ago. When he was alive, he lived at home, and his parents and siblings took turns providing for his care. They now actively grieve his loss.

Kevin's foster mother was his primary caregiver, and she was empathically concerned about his constant distress. Her even capacity at handling this distress was recognized as a truly remarkable caregiving gift and one that Kevin really needed. Her attunement to him was already high, and we spent time elaborating it by talking about her perceptions of his communications and validating them. I asked her, "What did it feel like to be in Kevin's skin?" She offered, "Nothing feels good, not for long anyway, and I cannot settle." I heard and validated what seemed like very reasonable readings of his frequent states. Taking my cues from her, I suggested that the first priority was helping him feel good and settled. She agreed. "Would this help her feel good and settled with him, also?" I wondered aloud. "Oh, yes, it would," she agreed. We worked together on swaddling, holding, and soothing attentively in response to his startle responses, tremors, and crying. I requested that she pay attention to his cues in response to these interventions and that she tune in to the kind of stimulation, holding, talking, looking, rocking, and so forth, that soothed him most and that he liked the most.

Kevin's foster mother discovered that he was very sensitive to sound and liked when people spoke to him in a soft voice. He was becoming familiar with her and oriented to the sound of her voice, tracked it, and gazed at her as she spoke to him or stayed within his range of vision. He was easily startled by sounds, too, and he averted his gaze if an unfamiliar person spoke with him. He was soothed by softly spoken words from a familiar person, by swaddling and by gentle rocking. He was beginning to recover from his lung condition and to tolerate his new formula much better. He was now able to take nearly 4 ounces of formula every 4 hours, and he was spitting up in lesser quantity. Kevin also liked his baths, and I suggested that his foster mother woo him and engage with him in the bathtub using the cues of his most liked activities. She touched and played with his chin, which he liked; she spoke with him softly and gently, and he gave her that slight smile more regularly.

Further suggestions included massaging his extremities—his feet and his hands—with the same connected, wooing approach for 15 minutes before his first quota of night sleep. Kevin's foster mother was interested in the suggestion. We discussed the basis for it and the way of implementing it. She asked if I would demonstrate it, and I did so on my own hands. Kevin's foster mother proceeded to rub the soles of his feet with a firm stroke, pulling up to his ankles and taut calves. He gave her a genuine full-face smile, the first any of us had ever seen. It was such a moment! We knew that he liked this and that it made him feel good, and we both commented as such. I spoke with him, gently narrating that I could hear him saying that he was feeling good and that his foster mother was doing this so that he could feel good more of the time. Kevin's foster mother pointed out that his extended limbs were relaxing. Kevin's arms and legs relaxed as she continued to massage slowly and firmly. I asked her if she could weave this into her daily routine before or after his bath prior to bedtime, and she was keen to do so. Because she seemed to like the intervention so much, I suggested that she try the same technique on herself or exchange massages with family members. I shared that I often did this and found it to be very relaxing. I also encouraged continuance of swaddling, holding, and gentle rocking as a way of soothing him when he cried and wooing, talking softly, and playing with him when he was awake and alert. I asked if she had enough help at home in coping with his excessive crying episodes, and she said that she could enlist her husband's help more. She said that Kevin really liked the sound of her husband's voice and that she would engage her husband in sitting in the rocker and gently rocking and holding Kevin when he cried. I encouraged her sensitive resourcefulness and her empathic connection with Kevin. She said that he mattered to her.

Kevin still cried loudly in distress when he was in discomfort, but the frequency and duration of crying episodes were much reduced. He was bonding with his foster family and recovered from distress in a few moments, 5–10 minutes most of the time. His reflux was significantly improved, and he was taking the nebulizer without trouble. His foster mother and he were enjoying their massage time together, and he was beginning to sleep better, feed better, and cry less. His tremors were still there, and both his foster parents were engaged in swaddling him, which managed and contained the tremors. He was beginning to track both his caregivers around the room from visual and auditory cues. He was tracking rattles and other toys offered to him as they were moved around near his face and upper body. I suggested adding a morning massage routine with energized strokes and demonstrated the same on my own hands. Kevin's foster mother agreed to try this.

"What does it feel like to be Kevin these days?" I asked his foster parents. "Oh, pretty good sometimes and pretty hard sometimes," said his foster father. "That is progress," I suggested, "big progress." They agreed. Kevin's foster father was saying that Kevin was now demonstrating a range of feelings and states and had moved on from his earlier intensely distressed restricted range. "What more is Kevin saying about his experience of himself in the world?" I wondered aloud, encouraging and elaborating his foster parents' connection with and empathy for him. His parents hesitated to elaborate, so I offered, "Maybe that he can rely on the voices and presence of two people in his life when he needs to be comforted, that feeding feels good, for the most part, and he can rest more." His foster mother joined in, saying that baths, massages, talk, play, swaddling, and holding all feel really good. "What about that hyperalert stare, though?" I wondered aloud. "What did that feel like in Kevin's skin?" His caregivers were puzzled and a bit stumped by my questions, but they tried to engage with them. I said that to me, he conveyed a facial expression indicating a touch of fear and a whole lot of stress and strain. I asked if this resonated with their experiences. His foster mother nodded, saying that he seemed so uncomfortable and stressed at times. I went on to comment on the fact that Kevin had a range of states now, and when he was not distressed or when he was bathing, he was more relaxed in his facial expressions, body tone, and posture. His foster mother expressed relief and gratitude that this was so, and his foster father nodded, sharing the sentiment with her.

Kevin was starting to orient to the bottle better and was sucking well. He was beginning to bring his hands to his mouth. Both these behaviors were helping him regulate. His foster mother's attunement and reading of his cues; her attentiveness, sensitivity, and responsiveness to his needs; and their developing relationship all were regulating him. His crying episodes were less frequent and less intense, and he was typically soothed in less than 20 minutes. His muscle tone remained hypertonic, though less so, and his movements were jerky. He remained sensitive to his environment, although he was not as easily startled by it. He arched back to communicate his need for less stimulation, and he interacted for brief periods of time in quiet, alert states with both his foster parents. His regional center referral for infant stimulation remained in process.

At this point 4 weeks later, I went deeper into dyadic regulation, asking Kevin's foster mother to observe her own breathing, which she did. I asked her to slow down and take deep breaths from her stomach, putting a hand lightly on her stomach as a way of guiding herself. I asked her how she felt, and she said she was more relaxed. I encouraged her to continue and to hold Kevin in her arms, look at him, speak gently, and keep steady with her slow belly breaths. I said that I would support them by doing the same and by introducing the sound of a Tibetan singing bowl. We tried this exercise for several minutes, and I introduced the soft, vibrating sound of a Tibetan singing bowl by playing it. The space acquired a quiet tranquility in which the sounds of the bowl and the synchronous deep breathing of the three of us took foreground. We continued for about 10 minutes, and then I asked Kevin's mother how she felt and what she had observed. She noticed how Kevin quivered at the first sound of the bowl and took in a big gasp of air, as children sometimes do after they have been crying hard; then his shallow breathing settled into a deeper rhythm that was in sync with hers and mine. She noticed that his facial expression became relaxed. I noticed that too. He did not have the hyper-alert stare. We continued to use this breathing–sound–attunement intervention in our twice-weekly sessions. Kevin's foster mother asked me if I had a recorded sound of the bowl, and I made her a copy on a CD. She began using that recording at bedtime, along with her massage routine. Both she and Kevin enjoyed slowing down and regulating their breathing with it. Slowly, the thus-far silent Kevin began vocalizing, to his caregivers' immense delight.

Less than 2 months after we had begun, it was time for closure. Kevin, now 5 months old, was establishing a good attachment with his foster parents. He anticipated their approach from hearing their voices, oriented toward them, discriminated their voices from those of others, and smiled often, experiencing and expressing pleasure. His foster mother was attuned to him and to his developing sense of himself in his skin. She successfully used her relationship with him and the tools of touch and sound therapy to center herself and to facilitate his experience of dyadic regulation. He had recovered from bronchiolitis and reflux with treatment and follow-up and was gaining weight well. He was still being monitored for his eyes, and he awaited regional center services for his motor development. He was to remain in this foster placement, as the question of long-term foster care versus adoptive care was taken up by the Department of Child and Family Services. In closing, Kevin and his foster family's joint accomplishments were highlighted and recognized through a process of joint narrative/storytelling in the therapy session. His foster parents realized and appreciated that they had come a long way together in a short time, and they were comfortable about seeking help again if they needed it. Kevin's foster mother said that "he was hard at first, but always a joy. Now he's simply a joy."

Kevin's Case and the Circles Framework

A brief discussion follows on the effect of the Circles framework in helping the clinician conceptualize and intervene in this case. In Circle One, Kevin's developmental functioning was observed and screened through available records and foster parent interviews. Regarding his socioemotional development, which was an area of relative strength, he did make eye contact but frequently averted his gaze, he did not break out into a social smile, he did not quiet easily when fed or comforted, and he did not recognize a primary caregiver or other significant caregiving adults. How could he have? He had experienced so many changes in these caregiving relationships already. Regarding his sociocultural identity, he is an African American male who had a very vulnerable start in life. His first chance at a stable start has been in his Hispanic American foster home. His foster mother is an aware, attuned, and caring person in these matters. She had a cloth rattle that had a brown-skinned, black-haired child's face on it. She had toys in his nursery that represented a variety of ethnicities and was aware of the fact that as Kevin grew up, he needed to see positive views of himself represented in the world around him. She encouraged visitations between his older siblings and him so that he could remain connected to his biological family and community. Both foster parents were responsive to empathically exploring and supporting Kevin's experiences in his skin and in the world through his communications about them (Lewis, 2000), and these discussions were supportively engaged in therapy.

In Circle Two, Kevin's attachment process had been disrupted on multiple occasions. It is impossible to know what he experienced in this regard in the first weeks of life. No one thought to record this attachment disruption in any hospital chart. We do not know the particular nature of his relationship with the older sister who initially stepped forward as his caregiver, but it is possible that the relationship did not go well, overall. From the disruptions of the attachment process, his in utero experiences, and his highly distressed state, we can safely assume that Kevin experienced multiple hidden traumas of caregiver unavailability and erratic attunement. He was adaptable and resilient, however, and responded well to the availability, regularity, and warmth of his foster parents. He especially needed their attentiveness when extended family visited and the house got loud and noisy. His foster parents were able to be sensitive to him and buffer him from the noisy environment by taking him to his own, quiet space when he needed it. They were also amazing in their capacity to handle his intense and prolonged crying in his early weeks of residence, a strength that was repeatedly recognized in therapy.

In Circle Three, the discussion did not go deeply into the foster parents' attachment histories, but neither did any roadblocks appear in our work that necessitated taking us there. Their observed capacities for availability, sensitivity, responsivity, and dedication spoke of positive histories and prognosis with Kevin, as well as their readiness to work with him. In Circle Four, a key issue was the family's grief over the loss of their developmentally delayed child. Their son was actively remembered and mourned in the family. The family said that they gained strength from one another and from their church in coping with their loss. Kevin's foster mother said that Kevin was not a replacement child but that being able to take care of him in their home meant that they were moving on with their lives. Nurturing young children, sustaining healthy relationships with family members, and giving time to take care of one another's needs were big priorities and values in this family and in its culture. Taking care of Kevin was right at the center of the nuclear and extended family's priorities.

In Circle Five, Kevin called to me as premature infants do. My native capacities for sensitivity and attunement aside, working through some of my own early experiences gets me energized to connect and help. It empowers me with a sense of agency, of knowing what to look for, how to make sense of it, and how to support those dealing with it. It gets me fired up about being there and about using fine-tuned empathic skills to help infants and their families connect and fit with one another. In Circle Six, my presence was easy, calm, and holding. I saw and supported, saw and followed, saw and cheered, saw and suggested, saw and guided. It was clear from the assessment data that regulation was a necessary point of focus for its effect on Kevin's relationship with himself, his relationships with the world, and his sense of well-being regarding both. I was aware that he had experienced many abrupt transitions and hidden traumas. I could see a beautiful, strong, but struggling infant. I could see the strengths in his orientation to his foster parents and their attunement and dedication to him. I could see that the foster family believed that helping Kevin was an important endeavor. My presence was affected by my awareness of all of these factors.

From Kevin's history and presentation, I noted multiple traumas, his ongoing physiological distress, restricted range of affect, and exaggerated, frequent startle indicating posttraumatic stress disorder. I also noted his hyperreactivity to stimulation expressed in excessive crying and motoric agitation, the hypertonicity of his limbs, and his fearful affect dominating and restricting his affective range, indicating regulatory disorder. The Special Start program tools (VandenBerg, Browne, Perez, & Newstetter, 2003) provided me invaluable help in thinking through the choices of regulators that I suggested for use at different points in the treatment with Kevin and his parents. I focused on attachment in the primary caregiving dyad by supporting and deepening attunement. I began to work with physiological/biobehavioral regulation around startle and tremors and with state regulation around crying. To facilitate these, I relied on physiological regulators (holding, swaddling, warmth, feeding, rocking) and relational regulators (wooing and identifying preferred sensory stimuli). As these targeted signs of dysregulation lessened, as caregiving attunement deepened, and as my rapport with the family increased, I turned my attention to motor regulation—his rigid tone, arm and leg extensions, and jerky movements—and to the state regulator—sleep and restlessness. Here, I used a combination physiological–relational regulator of attuned touch therapy or massage of extremities. Finally, as medical conditions improved through medical treatments and as feeding and sleeping improved and Kevin's crying lessened, I turned to deepening the foster mother's capacity for dyadic awareness, attunement, and regulation. Once again, I used a combination physiological–relational regulator of attunement, focusing on breath and sound. This regulator helped with the physiological regulation of breath and the state regulation (early emotion regulation) of hyperalertness and staring, bringing Kevin and his caregiver into more comfortable, secure, and relaxed states.

In 2 months, we had traveled a long distance, from working with a significantly and continuously distressed infant to working with one who was periodically and less intensely so, one who was able to enjoy life in his skin and communicate as much. This is the remarkable fact of early intervention—of how much important work can be done in very little time with informed and attuned knowledge and with developed capacity for presence. Intervention later in childhood and later in life, invariably, takes longer and costs more in every way.

In Circle Seven, the most pertinent parallel is my ongoing attention to self-care and self-regulation as a way of ensuring my own well-being, development, and fine-tuned state for undertaking such subtle work. Connection and attunement to family members and their relationships with Kevin and with one another—as well as the timing and staging of different interventions, particularly innovative ones—were supported by this attention to my own self-care. This self-care has included significant attention to the deep tranquility of breathing, and the practice of giving and receiving light at the dojo.

Research Bases That Assisted Me in My Work With Kevin: Hidden and Unhidden Trauma in Infancy and Early Childhood

As a clinician, my attunement to Kevin's condition was greatly enhanced through my study of the current research on how trauma is experienced in infancy and early childhood. A summary of this research follows, as a way of facilitating sensitization, conceptualization, and strategy formulation with traumatized at-risk and high-risk infants and young children such as Kevin.

Access to new ideas and technologies are allowing us to see beneath the affective, behavioral, and interpersonal expressions of trauma to its physiological and neurobiological substrates. The research and writings of Schuder and Lyons-Ruth (2004) lay out this complex picture involving the neuroendocrine system; autonomic nervous system; immune system; cognitive–behavioral system; and emotional, interpersonal, and coping systems. The subjective experience of trauma and intense fear arousal as well as the neurochemical response to it involves two main systems—

the norepinephrine–sympathetic–adrenomedullary system (NE-SAM) and the hypothalamic–pituitary–adrenocortical system (HPA). As Schuder & Lyons-Ruth point out, of these two systems, the HPA axis has been more widely studied because of the ease of access to its marker, cortisol, through noninvasive saliva swabs, whereas the NE-SAM marker, adenocorticotropic hormone (ACTH), is accessible only through a blood test. The HPA axis is a brain–body system that responds to perceived environmental threats by increasing heart rate and metabolism and reducing immune function, digestion, and growth. It prepares the body for fight–flight or freeze. Regulated functioning of the HPA axis is evidenced by a diurnal rhythm of cortisol that is high in the morning and low in the evening, turns up in response to stress, and then regulates and settles as the stress subsides. Dysregulation under stress is evidenced by hyperfunction (lack of return to a low level at the end of the day) or hypofunction (a flattening out of cortisol levels that can occur under enduring levels of severe stress). A developmental process is present in the establishment of rhythms, with infants demonstrating two cortisol peaks a day, 12 hours apart, that are uncorrelated with time of day. Within the first 3 months, and sometimes as early as the first 6 weeks, the morning peak begins to get established, and by the fourth year of life—parallel to the establishment of mature sleep–wake cycles—the diurnal cortisol rhythm gets established (Schuder & Lyons-Ruth, 2004). The safeguards of nature in our biology are fascinating to ponder. The human infant starts out life with large investments of time in sleep to support his intensive growth process. During this time, the immature, high-dose sleep patterns are supported by high-dose, two-peak cortisol rhythms. In the developmental progression of the infant, it is interesting to note the shift from higher rates of biological and psychosocial vulnerabilities (e.g., high infant mortality, child abuse, and neglect) and the more active HPA axis with a two-peak rhythm to lower vulnerability and a one-peak daily rhythm.

Schuder and Lyons-Ruth (2004) argue that the psychobiological study of trauma focusing on body physiology facilitates study earlier in infancy than the current attachment paradigm. It allows a glimpse into the neurophysiological experience of the infant and young child that can be at odds with what is apparent from external indicators of behavior. For example, Dozier and colleagues (as cited in Schuder & Lyons-Ruth, 2004) report incongruity in secure-looking behavior among foster children in the stressful situation of connecting with a foster parent and hypo/hyperresponsive HPA axis functioning. Such glimpses into the brain–body experiences of traumatized, at-risk children provide subtle early understandings and opportunities for early intervention for caregivers and professionals.

"In human infancy . . . experienced threat is closely related to the caregiver's affects and availability rather than to the actual degree of physical or survival threat inherent in the event itself" (Schuder & Lyons-Ruth, 2004, p. 70). Thus, a caregiver's emotional unavailability and/or interactive dysregulation and distressed affect are what Schuder and Lyons-Ruth aptly refer to as the bases for hidden traumas in infancy and early childhood. These traumas, subtle and easily missed without sensitization and orientation, can be powerful and enduring influences that contribute to early dysregulation of the HPA axis. They can affect the stress response system in a way that is similar to the effects of more obvious, less hidden traumas later in the life span. By affecting the structure of the infants' stress response system, traumatic experiences can reset the stress response system and, thereby, influence responses to subsequent trauma. Dysregulation in the functioning of stress physiology systems, as these authors indicate, is linked to adverse behavioral and emotional outcomes.

The scientific findings here advance, in an unprecedented way, our ability to know about and empathically connect with infant trauma. Imagine an infant such as Kevin in distress, dysregulated in sleep–wake cycles and feeding cycles. Imagine the infant's caregivers being fairly unattuned but well meaning and responsive. They respond to him readily, connecting with him at times, and not at all at others. They handle him with sensitivity, at times. The infant takes what he can get and calms down briefly when he receives some care and attention. But so much of the time in his skin in early and ordinary life is spent not at ease, not relaxed, not seen, felt, or secure. Consider next that this infant's experienced trauma, in a psychophysiological sense, may be very much at a par with an older child's or adult's experience of an obvious, massive trauma (e.g., a drive-by shooting of a family member, the destruction of a home in a natural disaster) but that he has very much more limited coping abilities and resources in dealing with it if he does not have attuned caregivers. The hidden traumas in infancy and early childhood are quite equivalent in effect, it seems, to bigger traumas later in life.

Consistent, emotionally available, connected caregiving that results in secure attachments seems to contribute to regulated HPA axis functioning and modulated stress response systems. Temperament seems to interact in interesting ways in this relationship between experienced trauma, attachment, and the infant's stress response system. Summarizing the findings of various studies, Schuder and Lyons-Ruth (2004) report that behaviorally uninhibited children, both secure and insecure, display the least physiological stress response activation. Behaviorally inhibited children who are insecure (avoidant and ambivalent) rather than secure have displayed such activation. Thus, inhibited, introverted, sensitive children who were exposed to hidden and multiple traumas in infancy and early childhood that resulted in insecure attachments may benefit from particularly attentive repairing and buffering of the quality and security of their caregiving relationships. Clinical evidence suggests that temperamentally reserved children may respond to trauma with withdrawal or with new or intensified fears, whereas temperamentally outgoing children may become defiant, aggressive, and risk taking. Young children can very often display both types of behaviors simultaneously in response to traumatic experiences (Lieberman, Compton, Van Horn, & Ghosh Ippen, 2003). The information on hidden traumas takes our clinical eyes, ears, and awareness to a new level of sensitivity, allowing us to detect and respond to traumatized infants and young children even before externalizing or internalizing behaviors are evident or before the goodness of fit in the caregiving dyad is greatly out of sync. Introverted and insecure children—those posing the least trouble in foster homes, day cares and schools—can be targeted for early intervention through professionals' training, sensitivity, and understanding of these children's needs and distress. In general, extroverted children and insecure, externalizing young children get the earliest identification and professional support. Introverted and insecure young children do not have the temperamental buffer that extroverted groups have; thus, their needs for early intervention call for empathic, early professional responsivity based on the research evidence.

Schuder and Lyons-Ruth (2004) report animal studies in which physiological mechanisms of caregiver proximity and presence, touch, milk, or nutrition as well as movement or rocking mediated the caregiving relationship, thus regulating stress response physiology. Of particular interest were studies by Myron Hofer (1973a, 1973c, as cited in Schuder & Lyons-Ruth, 2004), in which rat pups' heart functioning was regulated through nutrition (milk), and behavioral overactivity was regulated by the presence of a surrogate maternal figure. Although the application of these findings to human infants and caregivers is not yet clear, and much remains to be understood about how these mechanisms impact a developing infant's stress physiology, they are nonetheless fascinating to consider. Schuder and Lyons-Ruth also identify parallel social mechanisms, such as the child's ability to share affective states and signals and to use social referencing behavior, and the caregiver's emotional availability and capacity for interactive fit and regulation in communicating with the child.

From extensive and ongoing clinical and research evidence in the multicultural infant–family mental health field, we know that several important factors enable the caregiver to be sensitive, consistently emotionally available, and responsive to the child's psychobiology and the family's culture and context. First and foremost, balanced self-care and a history of the same in the caregiver are important in increasing sensitivity to one's own needs and cues as well as regulation of one's own states. Attuned relationships, willingness to be reflective, and adequate social supports can serve as resources for addressing and changing difficult attachment and self-care histories that are crucial to the improvement of intergenerational caregiving histories and outcomes. What is encouraging is that the willingness for undertaking this process can be highly successful. For example, in a longitudinal study, 30% of parents with childhood maltreatment histories who made such efforts, and who had had a caring adult available in childhood and a supportive partner in parenting, were able to break out of the intergenerational cycle of abuse (Erickson, 2005). Knowledge of child development that is culturally consonant and relevant, as well as realistic parental expectations that come from it, are also very helpful. Finally, as I argue in this book, an ongoing engagement in becoming fully present, alive and attuned in the moment, aware of subjective and objective information, is vital to nurturing new life and growth in relationships and families.

Innovative Interventions: Touch, Regulation, and Well-Being

Skin cells develop and are connected to the nervous system within 3 weeks after conception, making it the earliest developing sensory system (Zur & Nordmarken, 2006). The skin is also our largest organ and plays a major role in defining the boundary between self and other. It also contributes to preverbal and ongoing nonverbal experience of the world and communication with it. The skin is important to an infant's sense of ownership of the mother's body (Heller, 1997), made possible through attuned, sensitive caregiving that, in turn, contributes to containment, security, belonging, and well-being in the world. Research on touch has had prominent advocates such as Barnard and Brazelton (1990), Field (2000, 2001), and Montagu (1986). The evidence for the benefits of touch therapy/massage across a vast array of clinical conditions has been painstakingly demonstrated by Field and her associates (2000) at The Touch Research Institute in Miami, Florida. In newborns, particularly those with starts in neonatal intensive care units (NICUs), these studies demonstrate increased weight gain, better sleep, lower stress hormones, increased vagal activity, increased motor activity and alertness, and less fussiness. These outcomes fall into four categories of benefits (International Association of Infant Massage, 2005; Tayyib, 2006): (a) relaxation (balancing autonomic nervous system and stress hormone activity and regulating sleep–wake cycles); (b) relief (toning the digestive tract, aiding digestion, releasing endorphins); (c) bonding/attachment (experiencing positive, attuned, reassuring, and regular touch, thus releasing oxytocin and prolactin); and (d) stimulation (aiding the functioning of all major organ systems: nervous, circulatory, digestive, immune, and endocrine; Field, 2001). There is increasing evidence for positive outcomes experienced by mothers, fathers, caregivers, and extended kin in their own skins and in their relationships with infants and young children. This research evidence, integrated with evidence from the field, is summarized in Abbot (2005). The extensive evidence of benefits opens the way for further research illuminating the differential applicability of specific strategies and combinations of touch therapy with other sensory modalities such as smell (aromatherapy) or sound (music therapy) in specific conditions (Field, 2000).

Field (2001) has spoken extensively about the painful absurdity of no-touch policies in NICUs and has worked through various barriers to bring the benefits of massage to NICU babies; she has made this evidence available through the Touch Research Institute. Anthropologists have provided extensive information on low-touch and high-touch cultures and have associated these trends with different social outcomes, particularly with behaviors such as aggression (Field, 2001; Mead, 1935). In a multicultural society, we do, indeed, carry different cultural socialization experiences besides familial and personal ones to the use of touch in professional roles. In the context of psychotherapy, as well, there has been a long history and, perhaps, deep ambivalence to touch, with some variation across theoretical orientations. Studies have indicated greater use and openness among humanistic clinicians and greater suspicion and rigid avoidance among psychodynamic clinicians (Zur & Nordmarken, 2006).

Clinician orientations aside, young children force us to address this issue beyond any place of rigid avoidance, as only young children can do! Any clinician who works with this population has experienced a young child sitting on her lap, spontaneously touching her, or asking her for a hug. Such experiences do not offer easy escape to no-touch policies. Rather, the use of touch in a clinically sensitive, purposeful, and ethical way, respectful of clients' and clinician's cultural sensibilities, is a professional necessity and a responsibility. Preparation for this responsibility cannot be achieved through inflexible and unrealistic no-touch policies.

Touch is a powerful mode of communication, laden with meaning and rich with healing potential. Its professional use requires awareness and clarity that comes from professional preparation and self-awareness development on clinical, cultural, and relationship issues that affect it. Knowing one's clients, working with them respectfully and with informed consent, using good clinical judgment about timing, studying the research for current information, reflecting on client and personal experience in the work, being self-aware, and working within the scope of one's competence are all good guides in the integration of innovative practices, be they with touch or with anything else.

Innovative Interventions: Sound, Regulation, and Well-Being

Sound and breath are one, and practices of toning, chanting, and singing revitalize breath. . . . properties of sound medicine—entrainment, harmony, and homeostasis—represent the rational and spiritual foundation for a new movement in the healing arts and sciences.
—Gaynor, 2002 (p. 76)

The motivation for integrating touch therapy came from my experiences of growing up in a touch-oriented culture, experiencing massage routinely through childhood, personally knowing its benefits, and reading the extensive research on touch therapy that is currently available. The motivation for integrating sound therapy came from connecting with the work of a medical practitioner, Mitchell Gaynor (2002). This research is the work of an innovative, distinguished, and deeply compassionate medical practitioner who practices integratively and advocates for it. Dr. Gaynor's work was my introduction to Tibetan singing bowls. His attention to the psychosocial as well as medical aspects of his patients' healing process, his patients' very positive responses and outcomes, and the unfolding story of his own self-awareness development in his work are compelling for any health care practitioner. He works with a population of patients whose bodies are traumatized by life-threatening illness and whose minds, hearts, relationships, and families are traumatized with the news of it. He reaches out to them regularly, not only with the tools of conventional western medicine but also with the sound of Tibetan singing bowls and with the use of guided imagery. The sounds of the bowls, deep and resonant, are calls for centering and have been received by my clients, colleagues, and students very positively almost every time I have introduced them. At times, someone has expressed a preference for softer or louder playing. Only once, in my experience, has someone turned away and expressed a dislike of the sound, at which point I responded by stopping and returning to talk. Young children have invariably loved the playing of the bowls and so have their caregivers. The children have tried to play it themselves and figure it out. They have looked forward to the bowl-playing time, have identified me as the bowl lady, and have asked for the bowl when I did not produce it on my own. I have felt the spontaneous enthusiasm and joy that they have expressed as I have played. I have seen the sound regulate infants and young children, helping hypoalert children become more alert and hyperalert children become more relaxed. I have had their parents and caregivers say that they have felt calm, relaxed, and peaceful. I have heard students say that they have felt joy and expansiveness. As with any tool, it is less what it is and more how it is used that matters. As in the case of touch, attunement, empathy, respect for clients, sense of timing, manner of integration, personal familiarity, experience, and comfort with the tool are germane to its good integration into practice.

Gaynor describes the singing bowl in this way:

> *Whether made of brass and created by Tibetan craftsmen, or of crystal and manufactured here in the America, the singing bowls act as a medium in which our inner chaos and conflict can be re-configured into a sense of calm centredness through every cell of our body and mind. These remarkable vessels, as beautiful to behold as they are to hear, have become an integral and essential part of the sound-based guided imagery and meditation techniques that my patients and I use to resolve negatively charged emotions.*
> —Gaynor, 2002 (p. 107)

I use both the smaller metal bowls, which are easier to carry around but are harder to play, and the larger, more unwieldly crystal bowls that have to be handled with some care around young children but are much easier to play. Gaynor (2002) explains the benefits derived from the sound of the bowls with the principle of entrainment and extensive scientific literature that supports it. His explanation speaks to the inclination in all of nature for harmony, similar to the resonance between two pendulums in proximity that, sooner or later, begin to move together. Sonic entrainment leads the listener to resonate with the sound vibrations of the bowl at physiological levels (breathing slows); emotional–mental levels (feelings become more calm and positive; thinking is slower, deeper, and more organized); and cellular levels (sound travels through the water in every cell). This leads to greater homeostasis, physiological and biobehavioral regulation, harmony, and vibrancy.

Gaynor summarizes the research on sound as a healing modality by pointing out the two principal ways in which it works. The first way is by inducing relaxation and changing physiology (respiration rates, heart rates, blood pressure), and the second is through the experience of positive emotions and beneficial psychoneuroimmunological effects (decrease in stress hormones, increase in immune cell messengers and in endorphin release). Sound medicine, which has a long tradition of use in human civilizations, can facilitate early experiences of well-being in newborns and in new families by contributing to the balance and rhythm or regulation of their internal and interpersonal scaffold of experience and can set strong, healthy foundations for later development.

Questions

1. How would you summarize the clinical observations and conceptualizations in Kevin's case?

2. How would you summarize the clinical–cultural interventions in Kevin's case?

3. What have you learned about hidden and unhidden traumas that you can take away and apply to other cases?

4. What have you learned about the clinical–research interface and how advances in research can directly be brought to bear on what occurs in the clinical encounter?

5. What have you learned about the use of innovative interventions and about the considerations for integrating them into practice?

References

Abbot, S. C. (2005). *Comprehensive interventions for traumatized young children: Utilizing touch and smell to create somatosensory rich experiences which enhance development.* Unpublished PsyD doctoral project, Alliant International University and California School of Professional Psychology, Los Angeles.

Barnard, K. E., & Brazelton, B. T. (Eds.). (1990). *Touch: The foundation of experience.* Madison, CT: International Universities Press.

Browne, J. V. (2004). New perspectives on premature infants and their parents. *Zero to Three, 24,* 4–12.

Erickson, M. (2005, May). *My parents did that and I turned out fine, didn't I? Supporting families as they look back and move forward.* Keynote lecture presented at the California Council of Family Relations Annual Conference, California State University Northridge, Los Angeles.

Field, T. (2000). *Touch therapy.* Oxford, England: Churchill Livingstone.

Field, T. (2001). *Touch.* Cambridge, MA: The MIT Press.

Gaynor, M. L. (2002). *The healing power of sound: Recovering from life-threatening illness using sound, voice, and music.* Boston: Shambala Publications.

Heller, S. (1997). *The vital touch.* New York: Henry Holt.

International Association of Infant Massage. (2005). *The IAIM certified infant massage instructor's teaching guide.* Los Angeles: IAIM Press.

Lewis, M. L. (2000). The cultural context of infant mental health: The developmental niche of infant–caregiver relationships. In C. H. Zeanah (Ed.), *Infant mental health* (2nd ed., pp. 91–107). New York: Guilford Press.

Lieberman, A. F., Compton, N., Van Horn, P., & Ghosh Ippen, C. (2003). *Losing a parent to death in the early years: Guidelines for the treatment of traumatic bereavement in infancy and early childhood.* Washington, DC: ZERO TO THREE.

Mead, M. (1935). *Sex and temperament in three primitive societies.* New York: William Morrow.

Montagu, A. (1986). *Touching: The human significance of the skin.* New York: Harper & Row.

Schuder, M. R., & Lyons-Ruth, K. (2004). "Hidden trauma" in infancy: Attachment, fearful arousal, and early dysfunction of the stress response system. In J. D. Osofsky (Ed.), *Young children and trauma: Intervention and treatment* (pp. 69–104). New York: Guilford Press.

Tayyib, N. (2006). *From ancient tradition to modern clinical practice: Integrating touch/massage therapy into infant mental health, from birth to three.* Unpublished doctoral project, Alliant International University, Los Angeles.

VandenBerg, K., Browne, J., Perez, L., & Newstetter, A. (2003). *Getting to know your baby: A developmental guide for community service providers and parents of NICU graduates.* Oakland, CA: Special Start Training Program, Mills College, Department of Education. Retrieved January 24, 2007, from www.mills.edu/academics/grants_and_special_programs/specialstart/download/brochure_print.pdf

ZERO TO THREE. (2005). *Diagnostic classification of mental health and developmental disorders of infancy and early childhood: Revised edition (DC:0–3R).* Washington, DC: Author.

Zur, O., & Nordmarken, N. (Eds.). (2006). *To touch or not to touch: Exploring the myth of prohibition on touch in psychotherapy and counseling. Clinical, ethical, and legal considerations.* Retrieved December 22, 2006, from www.drzur.com/touchintherapy.html

CHAPTER 5
Identity and Difference: Mark "and I Don't Like That Brown"

Leena Banerjee Brown

Introduction

Mark was 3 years old when he began receiving mental health services in foster placement. These services carried him through his transition to reunification with his birth father. The modalities of play therapy (with child and clinician participating), dyadic therapy (with child, caregiver, and clinician participating), and family therapy (with child, caregivers, and siblings participating) were used in various combinations during different phases of the therapeutic process. The constant thread in the therapeutic process was the focus on relationships. The therapeutic work centered on Mark's emotional healing in the aftermath of multiple traumas. In the Circles framework, the focus translated to include his socioemotional development and his caregiving, sibling, and peer relationships as well as his sense of himself and his handling of differences with others. The integration of nurturing touch therapy, along with attunement (i.e., emotional availability, sensitivity, and responsivity), play, and other interventions focusing on relationships, was systematically demonstrated. Clinician self-awareness and self-care in the process of working on this case are also reflected upon.

Relevant History

Mark was 1 year old when he, his older brother Sid, and their two older half-siblings (a brother, Josh, and a sister, Jen) were removed from the care of their birth parents. At that time, the entire family was living in a van, and the children were unclean and fed erratically. Mark's mother had ongoing and untreated alcoholism. His father held a steady job in delivery, providing the family income and some bare necessities. At age 1 year, Mark was unable to sit on his own, stand, walk, or vocalize. He was petrified of taking baths, screaming at the top of his lungs as he was prepared for bathing. It was unclear whether this behavior was due to his being unused to taking baths or for some other reason.

Mark and Sid were placed in a residential care facility that accepted siblings together. Their half-sister and half-brother were placed in another state with their paternal grandparents, and Mark and Sid had monthly telephone call meetings set up with their siblings. These calls continued regularly and, on occasion, they exchanged drawings and photographs through the mail.

Upon arrival at the facility, Mark received medical attention for his severe diaper rash as well as a severe and untreated cold and ear infection. He also received infant stimulation services, which would help with muscle development and coordination, social interaction, vocalization, verbalization, and communication. He responded with enthusiasm and showed noticeable gains in the achievement of developmental milestones. Within 2 months, he had progressed from sitting steadily to taking first steps and confidently exploring his environment. He was enthusiastically vocalizing, making vowel–consonant sound combinations, combining gestures with words, and engaging attentively in interactions with his two primary caregivers. He enjoyed singing rhymes such as itsy-bitsy spider and playing interactive games such as pat-a-cake. Singing the alphabet song was a clear favorite.

The area in which he remained extremely fearful and resistant was bathtime. Dyadic therapy helped his caregivers and him in this area. Caregiver attunement around Mark's fear of baths was a focus of intervention. Therapists encouraged his caregivers to take him to his bath in a connected, nurturing, gentle way so that the experience of the bath could soothe him. As this work was proceeding and as his primary caregivers were paying special attention to their handling of Mark at bathtime, they found themselves shifting their attention and attunement in a similar way with Sid, as well.

Soon after this attunement, Sid shared an incredibly painful story with the primary caregiver at bathtime. His family was in what sounded like a motel room, and his mother, in an alcoholic stupor, tried to drown him in the bathtub. He managed somehow to slip out of her grip and escape from the bathtub. The primary caregiver asked who else was there at the time. Sid—who, by then, was sobbing in her arms—said that all his siblings, including Mark, were around. He said that their father was not there. He also said that he and all his siblings were crying and screaming at their top of their lungs.

The primary caregiver's sense of attunement to Mark's needs and his fears of bathtime deepened following these disclosures by Sid. In about 2 months, with his primary caregiver's sensitization and consistent responsiveness to his fears and need for extra reassurance during bathing, Mark was able to approach and experience bathing as a neutral event.

One year later, Mark and Sid successfully reunified with their birth father. The site social worker coordinated and followed up on the reunification plan and goals set up by the county social worker. These goals included the father's taking parenting classes, continuing to hold a steady job, and arranging a stable and adequate home and appropriate child care. The site social worker arranged transitional visits for Mark and Sid with their father and acted as a liaison between the residential program and the father. She followed up with the father and sons after the transitional visits, answering questions and giving developmental guidance. She also shared with him a summary of the clinical experiences in dyadic therapy with the primary caregivers and the recommendations that came from them and the clinician.

Needs and Strengths

Mark was a victim of childhood neglect. One year after reunification with his father, he was in out-of-home placement again, this time in foster care. His older brother had received a bruise on his back that allegedly had occurred at their babysitter's house. Their father had failed to follow up on it appropriately. This inaction resulted in both brothers being placed in foster care, with a new investigation and reunification plan. Their father remained committed to working on regaining custody of both sons.

At this time, Mark was 3 years old. As a Caucasian American boy, he had a round face, bright eyes, a pug nose, brown hair, and an incredibly endearing demeanor, at once full of mischief and warmth. He spoke nineteen to the dozen, and was fluent in English and Spanish. He was active, physically fit, and full of spunk. He loved the outdoors, especially playing in the park and on the jungle gym—climbing, swinging, jumping, and sliding adeptly at any chance that he got.

He was social in that he interacted with others, but he quickly became angry if something occurred that he did not like. For example, if a child wanted to join in a game he was playing with another child, he seemed to experience this event as necessarily disruptive and threatening. In these situations, he responded impulsively with immediate aggression as a way of expressing his feelings. He had a similarly difficult time sharing the attention of his foster mother. He physically tensed up in these situations, with his arm, chest, and shoulder muscles seemingly hair-trigger ready to act out; his facial expression and affect were also intense with defiance toward his caregiver as she encouraged him to share or as she set limits on his aggressive behaviors. At other times, he aggressively intruded in peers' play, particularly that of his older brother. These incidents of aggressive, defiant, impulsive expression of feelings in his social relationships occurred very frequently. The tenor of these relationships communicated patterns of interruption, disruption, and ambivalence. His foster mother described him as a "leader type who bosses others around," particularly his peers.

Mark's dreams were full of the themes of danger and threat, and he experienced these dreams three to four times a week. He was at an age when fears of various kinds, including nighttime fears, could be expected to increase. When he woke up and cried in his bed, his foster mother rose and went over to him to soothe him and help him return to sleep, which he did.

His 8-year-old brother, Sid, was also in the foster home. Mark looked up to Sid and was strongly bonded to this mild-mannered, protective older brother. In the foster home, they slept in the same room, on separate twin beds. He was impatient and aggressive with his older brother when things did not go his way. His older brother tended not to fight back immediately, but when Mark persisted with his aggressive behaviors, Sid responded in a similar fashion.

Mark was struggling to make sense of his early relationships. He was wondering in whom to repose his trust, his need for security, his need for belonging. He was wondering from whom he could get his cues in terms of who he was, where he belonged, how to express all of his feelings, how to treat others, how to deal with differences he perceived in others, and how to develop relationships with others.

He was placed with a foster mother who was a middle-aged Latino woman. He lived in a cozy, neat, and well-tended home with his older brother. He had a backyard in which he played and a neighborhood park that he visited regularly. His foster mother's adult daughter visited almost daily, and her two children (4- and 5-year-old boys) were being babysat at his foster home on weekdays while their parents worked. The family was bilingual and spoke both English and Spanish. Mark's father had twice-weekly monitored visits with his two sons. These visits occurred in the foster home, and the father kept most of these visits. Their birth mother had been absent from their lives for some time. After their initial removal from parental care, she sporadically showed up at monitored visits. She later stopped attending these visits and dropped out of her substance abuse rehabilitation program, as well.

Therapeutic Process: Observations, Interventions, and Outcomes

At the time of Mark's second placement in foster care, the county social worker made a referral for therapy. Home-based therapy services were set up through a community mental health program. In-home sessions were provided on a weekly basis, with the time divided between play therapy and dyadic and/or family therapy (first with the foster mother and foster family and, later, prior to reunification with the birth father, as well).

Phase I

Mark engaged with ease in play therapy, which took place in the room that Mark and Sid shared (with permission from all concerned). Sometimes Mark wanted to play on his bed, sometimes on the floor. He was enthusiastic about the individual time and attention from me, his clinician. He was very verbal and expressive in play and could symbolically communicate various themes such as fear, competitiveness, aggression, and need for warmth and security. He was also able to distinguish between reality and fantasy and move in and out of the two with ease. The theme to which he repeatedly returned, though, was that of fear.

Examples of this theme of fear and danger follow:

A teddy bear would meet a wolf. The wolf would want to harm the teddy bear but would not because God told him not to. The teddy bear was his father.

or

Barney, who was a very loving grandpa, would be walking along, and the wolf would suddenly appear. Barney somehow would be able to send this wolf away.

Despite the fact that Mark's stories invariably closed with safety, he continued to be tense and to work hard within himself to gain a full sense of that safety. The incongruence between the safety of his words and the insecurity of his feelings continued to be expressed in his body language.

Mark was gaining a sense of himself as a young boy, and he was identifying with his father. He was traumatized by his early experiences, and he persisted in holding on to the ubiquitous themes of danger and fear that remained faithful experiences in his life. As he reexperienced these fears, he repetitively played them out, both on his own behalf and on behalf of the main adult role model in his life, his father. He expressed this huge emotional burden in his play as well as in his physical bearing—a tense body with hair-trigger readiness to spring into aggressive, defensive action and push away the felt danger. He repeatedly expressed these emotions with increasing safety in the therapeutic relationship with me.

In the play, I inquired about his mother. Mark responded without skipping a beat. He said that his mother was hurt. He said that this made the teddy bear very sad, and as he felt this vulnerability on his father's behalf, he became overwhelmed with his own feelings, aggressively hitting and stomping the floor. He said, in his characteristic impulsive manner, that he was going to beat someone. I noted that he was very angry and that his stomping feet told me so. He agreed that he was. I asked him if telling me felt better than stomping his feet. He said it did; then he relaxed, sighed, and breathed more deeply.

In dyadic therapy, the initial focus was on helping Mark and his foster mother turn toward each other and connect around the nighttime fears so that he felt more contained and secure as he went to sleep each night. He tended to be tense in his body, even after his bath and bedtime story in his foster home. He now was not actively afraid of or resistant to having baths, but the tension and anxiety held in his body indicated that he may not have given up the fear altogether. He tended to be restless, tossing and turning in bed for at least an hour before he could go to sleep. At times, he would go over to Sid's bed and disturb him. Sid would patiently endure his brother's intrusions until their foster mother heard them, came back in to monitor the situation, and got Mark back into bed.

When asked by his foster mother if he liked their bedtime routine, Mark said that he did, that he liked both the bath and the storytime. His foster mother offered to take him to the public library every week, if he wanted, so that he could choose the books she read to him each night. He lit up at this suggestion. I asked the foster mother what she thought about the tension and tautness of Mark's body after a bath and before sleep. The foster mother said that she had a growing awareness of this state and wondered what to do about it. I suggested that the fear and insecurity that she was seeing expressed in play may have been emerging in this context, as well. I suggested that the foster mother give him a gentle back rub and hand and foot massage following the bath and storytime, if she and Mark were comfortable with this. The foster mother said that she would like to try this, and she asked Mark if he wanted her to. When he looked puzzled, the foster mother asked for his hand and massaged his palm. The clinician encouraged that the strokes be deep, not light and ticklish; that it be done for about 15 minutes; and that the gesture be done in a relaxed, emotionally present, and connected way. They practiced in the session, and Mark responded with a big smile. It was obvious that he liked this massage, and both he and his foster mother wanted to incorporate this activity into his bedtime routine.

Phase II

As Mark engaged in play therapy, he continued to tell stories about danger and fear and demonstrated defensive acts of aggression in play. He enjoyed reading books with his foster mother and with me on young children learning to cope with angry feelings. He continued to connect with deeply felt fears (his own, as well as his father's) and was ambivalent about his father's ability to protect him. He felt scared and angry about this situation. He connected with deep feelings of abandonment and anger toward his mother, feelings that he could hardly tolerate before lashing out with impulsivity and aggression. When he expressed these feelings in his play and stories, I remained highly attuned to them while listening, wondering, empathizing, and making sense of his messages. My foundation for understanding Mark's verbal and nonverbal communications included his history, my observation of his reciprocal relationships with significant others in family and social contexts, and my own relational experience with him.

As the therapeutic alliance deepened, Mark began to be more in touch with his own traumatic experiences and feelings. He not only expressed these feelings in play therapy, but he began to act out more against his foster mother, brother, and father. He became more of the bully and the "leader type." He gave his foster mother an increasingly difficult time with limit setting. He acted as though he was his own little man who did not need to listen to his foster mother and who needed to tell his older brother what to do, as well. His older brother, who typically did not stand up for himself, remained passive in response to Mark's bullying behavior. Mark was also into saying "no," but now his "nos" were very adamant and were occurring throughout his daily interactions with others. His demeanor and manner were serious, as though he meant business. His fears beneath the aggression obviously were affecting him. His relationship with me grew more ambivalent, as well. He would regularly say "I love you" to me, yet his interaction with me was more frequently challenging and defiant and occasionally distant. He was becoming accident prone and occasionally would regress, saying "I am baby" and then speaking like one. Throughout these behaviors, I held an unvarying, warm, and accepting presence toward him.

At this time, the therapeutic strategy moved to the inclusion of family therapy, as Mark himself was pushing the therapeutic container of the dyadic relationship to expand to the container of the family system. He was increasingly becoming a management challenge in the family, and the whole system needed to be addressed. There were now three layers of therapy at work: (a) play therapy for about a half hour (and Mark continued to engage in it with enthusiasm); (b) dyadic therapy for another half hour with Mark, his foster mother, and his clinician; and (c) family therapy for the second hour.

In the dyadic work, the focus was on helping the foster mother enable Mark to express his feelings. She was coached to identify interactions or events from earlier in the day in which Mark had been angry, sullen, or aggressive and then talk with him about this behavior and ask him about his feelings.

As he identified his feelings, she was coached to respond with understanding and to praise him for expressing these feelings. I introduced the foster mother and Mark to the feelings chart, and they enjoyed identifying and labeling feelings as well as telling stories about those feelings. Mark seemed to be most happy having the opportunity to receive positive, undivided attention from important adults in his life. He also was soothed and uplifted by the feelings of being understood, heard, seen, and nurtured in these ways. He was a bright and socially oriented boy by nature, and these positive experiences contributed toward him relaxing his body posture and smiling with dancing eyes. At the same time, the bedtime routine was continuing to work well, and Mark was reporting significantly fewer nightmares or "bad dreams."

In family therapy, the foster mother was supported in her executive/leadership role in the family. The goals were helping her set limits with Mark with greater ease, facilitating conflict resolution between Mark and others, helping Mark be less intrusive with others, and teaching Mark about being respectful of her authority. She was supported in continuing to build a relationship with Mark's birth father during his visits, sharing the importance of all these issues, and discussing both successful and unsuccessful strategies. She was also assisted in working on Sid's need to engage more, to stand up to his brother, and to get help from her when this strategy was not working. The clinician continued to affirm to Mark and his brother that their foster mother was in charge of them and was the one whose rules counted until they returned to their father. Then, their father would once again be the one in charge. As the executive system in the family worked on accomplishing the complex tasks of routine caregiving and emotional healing for the foster children, the children were gaining the emotional freedom to be more carefree and to experience their respective childhood ages of 3 and 8 years. In one family session, I brought up the theme of expressing feelings and said that all feelings were fine, but actions that hurt others were not. The foster mother nodded, Sid listened, and Mark began to tense up his body and tighten up his face. I encouraged the foster mother to see him, attune to him, and ask about his feelings. When he said that he felt angry, I modeled for the foster mother by telling Mark that all of his feelings were OK, but hurting someone else with his angry feelings was not. Then, I leaned over and asked if he might like his back rubbed. He nodded, saying "yes," and I gently but firmly stroked his spine up and down. The foster mother and I watched how Mark began to relax his body posture, breathe more slowly, and regulate the intensity of his strong emotions in response to the touch and nurturing support. His foster mother took over from me in a very natural way and praised Mark for sharing his angry feelings and for not biting or kicking anyone. He smiled a wide, quiet smile, as did his brother. I asked if Mark could ask his foster mother for such massages at times. He smiled impishly and said "no," and then he added that he could call it a "sausage" and ask for that sometimes. I replied that "sausage" could be a great code word for "massage," and as long as he and his caregivers knew it, it could work very well.

At one family session at lunchtime, I stood by Mark as the family, along with the visiting grandchildren, settled in for lunch. One of the grandchildren asked the clinician several questions that she proceeded to answer. She noticed that Mark was beginning to get tense. His body language and his facial expression were beginning to indicate that he was resenting this attention that the clinician was giving his peer. I asked if he had any feelings that he wanted to speak about. Mark said that he did, that he was angry and that he wanted to sock the grandson. He proceeded to point at the grandson's face and said, "and I don't like that brown." Looking at all the brown faces in the room (including mine, South Asian American and darker skinned), he continued pointing at each one of them, saying, "and I don't like that, and that, and that brown either."

The foster mother stood in shocked silence. I mustered the courage to proceed and said, "But, Mark, your hair is brown." He seemed to ignore me. His affect and facial expression clearly communicated anger and rage. He said that his father, who was very strong, would come and sock that boy. I continued to speak as the grandson, who already looked scared, started to cringe a little; the foster mother was still stunned and speechless. I said that I thought that strong people never had to hurt anyone and that they could love everyone. This is what made them strong. Mark took a long, deep sigh; it seemed as though he had breathed a sigh of relief. His taut body started to relax. I noticed that my comment seemed to have made sense to Mark. The tension that had mounted up in the room began to dissipate. I then leaned over close to Mark and said, "You sometimes get so mad, don't you?" He nodded and started tearing up. I put my arms around his shoulders. His foster mother came over in a few minutes and put her arm on his shoulder, too, and I slowly moved away.

Phase III

Mark began to become very interested in the garden. The sessions were now divided between play therapy and family therapy. During play therapy, he and I would take walks in the garden, talking about growing things. Mark had great interest in plants and flowers, bugs, butterflies, and trees. He wanted to share his flower and leaf collections with the others in the home, most of all with Sid. He treasured, with extraordinary gentleness and care, any little flowers or interestingly shaped twigs that I found and gave him. He made up songs that expressed his happy feelings. A whole other side of his person was becoming alive. His positive experiences in the family were steadily increasing. He followed a preschool-like curriculum with his foster mother and was preparing to return home with his father. He respected his foster mother and was rarely, if ever, defiant with her. Sid was the only one whom he occasionally tried to bully, but his foster mother had learned how to intervene and help Sid do a better job of finding his own voice in these situations so that they were better managed.

At this point, reunification was nearing, and the family sessions began including Mark's father. His father initially had a difficult time following Mark's cues the way that the foster mother did. He was open to learning, and, by and large, he progressed well. He also was being helped by the county social worker with preschool arrangements for Mark. He, himself, had put into place some additional babysitting arrangements in preparation for his sons' return. Mark soon minded his father as well as he did his foster mother. He was sleeping restfully, and his aggression was very much in check. He remained prone to periodic displays of aggression when he was especially tired or not feeling well. But his caregivers were very aware of where he was coming from and how to help him.

He responded very well to nurturing touch, and the foster mother taught his receptive father how to nurture him in this way. Initially, when his father massaged him, Mark curled up like an infant, assuming a fetal position and vocalizing like an infant in his father's arms. His father recognized what was happening and held Mark closer. After a few times, Mark no longer regressed in this way. His father seemed to greatly enjoy the chance to massage and relax Mark, who, in turn, enjoyed the experience. Mark's father would often say, "I didn't know that he needed that," intimating that he gladly would have given the massage before, had he known.

Mark's father opened up, too, and I spoke with him in the absence of the others. He described his own early deprivations, his hopes and dreams of going to college to actualize his potential, and his inability to do so. He mentioned that his father and mother instilled in him a work ethic but that his childhood was emotionally barren for him. His father was hardly ever there, and when he was, he was remote. He had an unpredictable temper and was physically punitive. His mother provided the basics of care in the home but was not emotionally demonstrative. He was bright and wanted to seek higher education; however, the family was poor, and he did not know how to go about realizing his hopes for himself. He eventually drifted away from his family, moving to the Midwest, and began working in low-paying jobs, keeping alive his love of learning by reading voraciously in his spare time. Mark's father was psychologically minded and felt motivated to help his sons. The clinician strongly recognized him for these qualities. She encouraged him to seek the support and process of individual therapy so that he could work through his own pain and disappointments. She suggested that this therapy could help him raise his children successfully and have a new start in his own life. He agreed, and a referral and linkage were made prior to reunification. I asked how he felt about his relationship with me in therapy, given that we were people of different colors and cultures. He said that he felt very comfortable in therapy, that he felt he could be really open, and that he was being helped. He was also able to say that he had grown up with the message that people who were different were not to be trusted. I offered that Mark may have gotten that message, too, and shared a summary of the incident that spoke to this experience. I explained what had happened, and the father listened. Silence followed. It was not an especially uncomfortable silence but one indicating that the father was taking things in. I left it at that.

The family therapy process (which included the father) proceeded well. However, Mark had an outburst in a session when the transition to reunification with the father was brought up. Transitions were scary for Mark. The foster mother assisted Mark's father in encouraging him to express his feelings instead of stomping his feet, falling to the ground, or throwing his book down. Mark told his father that he was angry and that he would kick him. His father responded swiftly, saying that Mark could not belong in his family if he behaved in that way. Mark dissolved into tears. I stepped in to help renarrate with the father. I encouraged him to reach out to Mark. He did, and eventually he had Mark in his arms. I suggested that the father did not want Mark to hurt anyone when he was angry and that he did not want anyone in his family to hurt anyone. I said that Mark was his son and would always be a part of his family, no matter what he did. His father nodded his head affirmatively and apologized to Mark for hurting his feelings. He said that Mark was his son, that he loved him, and that he would always be part of his family.

Just prior to actual reunification, Mark had another intense outburst in family therapy. He had an aggressive tantrum that was worse than those he used to display. He fell to the floor, threw books and toys all over the room, and screamed and cried until his father picked him up, held him, and began stroking his back and his hands very gently, speaking with him in a quiet tone. As his father held him, he said that Mark was afraid of returning home and being abandoned by him again. Mark became very still and calm as he heard his father read his behavior. He had been deeply understood by one of the most important people in his life.

Soon after this incident, Mark had a dream. He dreamt that he had a big dog with six puppies. The dog and the puppies were all very loving and playful with him, and he was full of joy as he spoke of them. I encouraged him to draw his dream, which he did. He later put the drawing up on the wall by his bed to reinforce his feelings of hope and of not feeling alone and abandoned.

A few more sessions of exchange and preparation were conducted as a way of facilitating the move from the foster home to the father's home. I scheduled follow-up sessions after the reunification to provide support to Mark, Sid, and their father following the transition. The boy who went home had done a great deal of work and a great deal of healing, as had both his families. His father informed me that he had a sense that Mark was really strong and really bright and that, if things fell right for him, he could do a lot with his life. This seemed like a reasonable hope.

Reflections Using the Circles Framework

Circle One: Development

At 3 years of age, Mark was on target in terms of physical, cognitive, language, and communication development. These were areas in which he was delayed at age 1 year when first placed out of home. He was very responsive to infant stimulation services at that time, and he overcame his motor and language delays, thus demonstrating that these delays were clearly a result of neglect and deprivation of adequate attention, interaction, and nurturance. Mark grew to become a talented child who was active, well coordinated, and had promise, perhaps, as an athlete. He was bright and communicative, and he had a strong vocabulary and expressive ability.

He was equally responsive to dyadic therapy, responding to the sensitivity, attunement, responsiveness, and compassionate touch of his primary caregiver to overcome fears and anxieties at bedtime. However, he continued to be prone to fear and anxiety as well as difficulty handling such feelings when they turned to anger. These feelings regularly got in the way of his interactions and relationships with caregivers and with peers. These feelings appeared in therapy as themes that he visited repeatedly through play and storytelling. He was able to engage well in play, use words and gestures to express deep and complex feelings, distinguish reality from fantasy, and move with relative ease between the two. He opened and closed successive circles of communication in play and in conversations outside of play. Nevertheless, he regularly got stuck with the intensity of painful feelings inside of him. He felt fear, danger, injury, and anger, not only in his mind but also in his body. His expressive face, words, and body postures told this story as his clinician listened. When he was contained, as he was in therapy, he became manageable and responsive to being seen, felt, and understood. When he was on his own or not in a relational container, he lost impulse control by acting out his feelings with aggression and becoming socially disruptive.

Regarding his sociocultural identity, Mark had established a sense of distrust in relationships in the world. This filled him with fear and anxiety that, at times, turned into anger and angry behavior. In light of his history of possibly witnessing the near drowning of his older brother, he may have experienced moments of deeply felt terror that typically remain embedded in implicit preverbal memory. He had not established basic trust in relationships but seemed not to have given up on trust altogether, and he was ambivalent about it. Therein lay his resilience. He was responsive to the nurturing of substitute caregivers, but he did not trust them enough to accept their limit setting. He did not trust them to really keep him safe. Because of his lack of experience, he did not know that to explore the world successfully and to develop autonomy, one has to be able to explore it safely.

He found himself and his family to be an ethnic minority in his surroundings. As a young child, he was at the age when he was capable of categorizing observations as similar and different. His life with his family had been hard on physical, emotional, and economic levels. They were socially isolated, yet at the same time, via the media, he had the opportunity to be exposed to his White majority position in society. He observed that there were many others who looked, spoke, and seemed like him and who seemed to enjoy many things, could do many things, and had much to say. Yet his father stood in contrast to these media images. He conveyed shame and disappointment rather than served as a model of hopeful identity and an anchor of stability.

In moments of deeply felt inadequacy and fear, which were inevitable experiences for Mark as he grew close to another human being, he projected his intense fears and feelings aggressively. In the previously described situation in therapy, at such a moment of felt inadequacy, he became verbally aggressive and attacking about differences in color between him and his Latino foster family and Asian American clinician. His behavior may have been influenced by exposure to the modeling of his father or others in his history. My holding of his attack, and its associated derision and pain, offered him a new and positive perspective and reached out to him across the divide of color, helping reconnect him to a place of comfort within himself and a place of openness toward his foster family and clinician. My interventions enabled him to move from fearful anger, aggression, and isolation toward a more trusting connection through which he could release sorrow and gain hope.

Circle Two: Caregiving Relationships

The quality of Mark's caregiving relationship with his mother was presumed as very inadequate. His words and actions in play therapy revealed that he felt abandoned by her and angry toward her. He also felt his father's disappointment and sadness in his loss of her. Mark conveyed these feelings in play, speaking with deep sadness about his mother being hurt and out of his reach and about his father's sadness around this. As he connected with these feelings, his sadness turned to anger, and he aggressively stomped the floor. His mother was alcoholic, allegedly abusive to family members and, one can imagine, only erratically available to him. His father, who earned the family a very modest but regular income, was absent most of the time during Mark's infancy. Thus, Mark's development was delayed as a result of pervasive neglect.

Mark went on to experience changes in primary caregiving as he was placed in residential care that provided continuity in his interactions with his father and sporadic contacts with his mother. He was responsive to caregivers who were attentive to him. He responded well to the regularity and predictability of the structure of his relationships with these caregivers and worked through some intense fears around bathtime in these relational contexts.

He reentered foster care at 2.5 years of age and was warmly received by his foster mother. He was responsive to her but possessive of her attention. Just as he was loathe to share his toys (an age-appropriate impulse), he was particularly unwilling to share her attention. The sense of insecurity that he expressed in his relationship with his foster mother was much more deeply embedded in his relationship with his father. Mark was attached to him. His face lit up like a lightbulb every time he anticipated his father's visits. He spoke of his father frequently between visits. He looked up to him and looked forward to his time with him. But he was insecurely attached to him, ambivalent about how close to get to him, easily threatened, and easily anxious if something did not go smoothly or did not go his way. Mark needed his father, but he was not ready to have him back in his life, and who could blame him?

Circle Three: Primary Caregiver

Mark's father, Hugh, had his own history of early privations, as well. His father was a fearsome character who was mostly absent, and his mother was undemonstrative and distant. Hugh was a very bright person who had hopes and dreams of attending college and achieving many things, but he had almost given up. He was very tall, heavyset, untidy, and uncaring in the way he dressed. He spoke well and could be articulate and engaging. He had some knowledge of childhood development, his expectations of his children were fairly realistic, and his interest in learning more was genuine. He maintained his delivery job and appeared to like it. He had no family or social support whatsoever and was unclear and hesitant about developing these support systems. The therapeutic process was instrumental in his building a bridge with the foster mother; establishing a good, supportive relationship with the clinician; and agreeing to develop a similar one with another clinician who was working with him on issues in his own childhood and present life. Other suggestions, such as becoming active in social activities at his church or in single-parent groups, were not of interest to him. But Hugh was willing to consider becoming active in a community sports league in which he could enroll his two very eager sons after reunification.

Circle Four: Family Relationships

Mark grew up in a family in which the power and authority structure worked partially and inconsistently. His father, Hugh, had sustained jobs and consistently had tried to earn a living, but he was hardly present at home. Hugh provided for the family, but the family had no roof and no adequate or regular meals or care. Mark's mother had a substance abuse condition and was in deep, untreated, and unresolved anguish of her own. It seemed that the children's day-to-day existence and needs were left to chance and to themselves. The message that Mark may have gotten from his parents during his infancy was that he could not rely on them to care for him, nor could he count on their competency in steering the family on the road of everyday life. His parents' authority over him and his siblings was taken away twice in his early years as a result of this situation. Thereafter, his mother abandoned the family and her responsibilities. Fortunately, primary caregivers in Mark's early out-of-home residential care facility and his last foster mother provided positive models of adequate executive functioning in parent–child relationships. Mark seemed compelled to step in and take charge in relationships, especially during times of stress. His caregivers had to help him be a 3-year-old, thus allowing him to ease off from these emotional burdens to which he was unconsciously prone and to let his foster mother take charge instead.

Mark was prone to overfunction; he tended to invert the executive hierarchy/authority structure when he was stressed and when he was in touch with his unresolved fears and anger and with those present in the interpersonal context. The boundaries in his early family relationships had been diffuse and enmeshed. His parents had shared too much of their fears and helplessness with him. He had responded with empathic feelings for them and was sensitized to their needs, but he was helpless to help them.

Mark was very close to his brother, but he also frequently and regularly intruded in his brother's space, his possessions, and even his body (pulling him into knock-down, drag-out fights in which Mark acted out his aggression while his brother tried to keep him at bay until help arrived). He was similarly enmeshed in his relationship with his father. Mark was overwhelmed by having to cope with his own sadness, anger, and powerlessness as well as by trying to embrace his father's equivalent feelings.

The sequences of interactions in his relationship with his foster mother around his nighttime fears seemed to have been appropriate and responsive. However, he needed even greater sensitivity as he was reexperiencing old wounds of abandonment as well as lack of a stable home and caregiving after his second removal from home. Therapeutic facilitation of attunement and the introduction of compassionate, nurturing touch helped meet his emotional needs for safety, security, and reassurance.

Their family developmental structure and life cycle were continually being reconfigured because of the changing realities of the experiences of Mark and his family. Mark's birth parents faced the challenges of rearing young children in a blended family in poverty and of remaining connected through successive reconfigurations, something at which they succeeded only partially. Mark and Sid's family structure went from an underresourced blended family to out-of-home residential placement with separation from half-siblings to an underresourced, single-parent family to a foster family to a more fortified, reunified, single-parent family. The challenges of adjusting to all of these changes within the first 3.5 years of life was exacerbated by a multitude of losses—a family that could no longer live together, loss of the mother, half-siblings living out of state, and loss of trust in the father's care. What remained steady were the father's presence and commitment to improve his ability and record of caring for his sons together. The nurturing and relatively stable experiences of caregiving from primary caregivers and from the foster mother also likely contributed to trust and positive expectations in relationships.

Mark was Caucasian American. He was of fourth-generation Eastern European American stock on his father's side and Anglo American on his mother's side. His father had moved away from his family, keeping minimal contact with them. He believed in God and infrequently attended church. He told his children to believe in God, to pray every night, and to believe in God's protection. He became a member of the working poor. The family's life was one of financial insecurity, of living hand to mouth, of having only the bare necessities only at the best of times. The father bought junk food regularly for his children, but when the foster mother and clinician gave input to the father regarding nutritional ways of eating, he was responsive and replaced junk food treats with strawberries and grapes. When they had a roof over their head, the family lived in poor neighborhoods. Their community was predominantly Latino. Mark's father, Hugh, spoke of his neighbors with a tone of "otherness" and disdain. He referred to "those people" who lived in overcrowded families and who dirtied the city streets. Paradoxically, he felt very comfortable with the care "they" gave their children and sought out his neighbors to babysit his children. He believed in having a tidy, clean, and organized home with separate spaces for adults and children, separate beds for his sons, and enough room for playing, but he admitted that he rarely had the physical or emotional energy to follow through as a parent and make all of these things happen.

As a man, Mark's father seemed weighed down by his own unexamined shame of not realizing the dreams he had for college and not using what he referred to as "the potentials of his mind." His shoulders drooped, he dressed without care, and he would slink around like he wanted to hide. This behavior was ironic, given his significant size and stature. He had hopes for his children that he clearly needed to separate from any vicarious needs of his own for personal fulfillment. For example, when Mark said that he wanted to be an ice cream man, his father quickly and reactively countered that he would make a good doctor or scientist. Intergenerational patterns on Mark's paternal side—which have influenced his vulnerability for deeply felt inadequacy, proneness for abandonment, and resilience to keep trying without giving up—are worthy of exploration, discovery, and reflection. These patterns contained within them high levels of fusion as well as cutoff and potential for differentiation. Engaging with, reflecting upon, and working through these patterns would contribute to Mark's father being happier in himself, happier as a parent, and more able to pass down strengths to Mark and his brother. At the same time, it is important to acknowledge that this information and analysis does not include the engagement or data from Mark's maternal side, which, in a more optimal situation, would be available and included.

Circle Five: Clinician's Reflections

As a clinician, I felt an immediate draw toward Mark. Upon reflection, I realized that his face bore a strong resemblance to that of one of my own sons. It was going to be easy to connect with him; however, my connecting with him needed to be balanced at all times with my overreaching the empathy into identification while appropriately connecting with his parents, sibling, and peers with whom the work was also occurring. These reflections and elements of self-awareness were critical in carrying me through moments when the therapeutic encounter became intense.

Mark's verbal assault on me and others on the basis of color took me completely by surprise. I was aware that he was able to categorize and label colors and that he most likely had absorbed the similarities and differences in color of those around him. His angry affect and demeanor made his statement about color feel like an act of violence. Perhaps that is why I made the connection in my mind about strength in nonviolence. The fact that Mark could resonate with that connection was no surprise to me. He was in touch with his capacity to love and be loved, to connect and be connected to, to understand and be understood. I had experienced this with him over and over again. He had reason to distrust others, but through the therapeutic process, he was wholly engaged in a struggle at learning how to repose his trust in them, and he was making progress.

Circle Six: Clinician Presence

I felt that much was asked of me as a clinician in this case, and, equally, that much was given to me to work with. There was a high level of energy and hope that were constantly present in the work despite the complexities and intensities of the challenges that needed to be faced. Mark experienced a series of severe stressors in his first years of life. Inconsistent, neglectful care in infancy left him delayed in multiple developmental domains. It seems likely that he experienced at least one highly charged traumatizing event during this time, that of the attempted bathtub drowning of his older brother by his drunken mother. He further experienced removal from home at 1 year of age and again at 3 years of age. In thematic play, Mark repeatedly expressed his anxieties and fears, which transformed into anger and aggressive behavior with daily regularity. He had experienced intense fear of taking a bath and falling asleep. His affect and his body language were entirely consistent with his chronic anxiety and aggression. He experienced difficulty in peer relations, in sharing caregiver attention, and in sharing space and toys, and invariably he became anxious and aggressive in these situations. The diagnosis of posttraumatic stress disorder was applicable.

All of the therapeutic work was done in a relational context in light of Mark's age and according to the standards of practice associated with it. The modalities of play and dyadic and family therapy were used in differing combinations throughout the process. As therapy unfolded, my understanding and connection with the clients grew. From this understanding came a sense of connection with the flow and pulse of the therapeutic process as a whole. The timing and choice of therapeutic modalities was guided by my connection with the clients and knowledge and experience with the Circles domains. In retrospect, it is clear that these decisions and actions took the therapeutic process through three phases.

In Phase I of the therapeutic process, the dyadic work was supplemented with individual play therapy because of Mark's ability to engage very well in representational play and because of the depth of his traumatic history, which had a far deeper reach than his relational history with his current caregiver. These two elements enabled me to directly explore, listen, and understand Mark's story, resiliencies, and needs. I integrated these experiences as a central aspect of not only play therapy but dyadic therapy, in which Mark's foster mother increasingly became emotionally attuned to him.

In Phase II, Mark began to establish trust and safety in his foster home. In therapy, he became increasingly in touch with his painful feelings of anxiety, fear, and anger. This connection resulted in an increase in acting out in the family context and, thus, the need for incorporating family therapy. The therapeutic container was expanded from the relationship with Mark to the relationship with Mark and his foster mother as well as the inclusion of the foster family as a whole. Key struggles emerged and were worked through in play, the dyad, and the family.

In Phase III, the consolidation of strengths and preparation for transition back to the father's home were undertaken in the dyad and the family. At this time, family therapy included key exchanges between the foster mother and birth father, thus facilitating the transition process and extending the therapeutic container from the present home to the new one. Key struggles emerged between Mark and his father in preparation for reunification, and I provided guidance and facilitation in this process.

Touch therapy was integrated into the dyadic and family therapy experience at several key points. Attunement to Mark's acute and physically held stress led the way, and his immediate positive response and relaxation indicated the helpfulness of the effort. I was empathically attuned to his body language that expressed anxiety, fear, and anger. I reached out with words of understanding and with nurturing, compassionate touch that served to strengthen the connection; release his anxiety; and increase his regulation of breathing and emotions, relaxation, and trust in his caregiving. Teaching his foster mother and birth father to massage his extremities and back was, thus, very helpful. His father's initial use of touch caused Mark to experience poignant regression and to working through felt deprivations. His father's availability and responsiveness were equally poignant and were integral to Mark's healing process. It was as though they were making up for lost time. Mark responded well to connected, nurturing touch by letting his guard down, relaxing, and regulating the intensity of his emotions.

Circle Seven: Self-Care

Maintaining client confidentiality at all times, I found it necessary to occasionally share some of these experiences with selected colleagues as a means of gaining perspective and support. These communications and ongoing self-care practices were essential in helping me go with Mark and his family to the deep places of intense emotion that were visited in this therapeutic process. Self-care practices, for me, included meditation, walking, reflection, reading, study group membership, supportive collegial relationships, time with family and friends, and laughing with my own children. This experience of self-care helped me to allow painful, provocative feelings into the therapy room, to experience these feelings with Mark and his family, and to hold a supportive space as they worked through them. This self-care further enhanced my sense of timing in offering Mark and his family suggestions for moving forward, recognizing and validating their gains, and strengthening their motivation to ask for professional help in the future if they needed it.

Questions

1. *How would you describe Mark, developmentally, at the point of his second reunification with his father and brother? How would you sum up his strengths and his needs? How would you follow up on your assessment? Would you use therapeutic modalities? If so, which ones? Would you make other service linkages, community resource referrals, or other resource recommendations? If so, which ones?*

2. *If Mark's father requested continued family therapy after reunification, what issues would you focus on, and what approach would you take? If you were to do a genogram, would you explore the issue of father's engagement and clarity with his own life goals as a parent and as a man? Could this be instrumental in promoting healthy parenting behaviors and preventing vicarious expectations of Mark and Sid?*

3. *What alternative, productive ways come to mind for dealing with the issues of sociocultural identity and differences that came up in family, dyadic, and play therapy? How could engagement with these issues be further supported from a mental health promotion and prevention standpoint in the pre- and postreunification phases of the therapy?*

4. *How do you think the therapeutic work, in this case, was affected by the clinician's female gender? How could the situation have changed with a male clinician?*

5. On the basis of your theoretical orientation(s) and experience in practice, would you use all three elements of play, dyadic, and family therapy in this case? Why and why not? Would you use them in similar/different combinations at the different phases?

6. Mark communicated vividly through his play and through the imagery in his stories and dreams. As you reflect on what he said through these stories and dreams, which of his experiences, transitions, and transformations stand out for you, and why? How might your insights organize or mobilize you to act if you were in the role of clinician for him and his family?

7. Identify and reflect on particular moments in the therapy that stand out for you when the clinician was present and attuned with Mark and members of his family. Articulate your understanding of what occurred in those moments, the clients' presentation, the clinician's presence, the interventions, and the client feedback. Repeat the exercise for moments in which the attunement seemed less in sync to you, and articulate the dynamics that occurred. If you were in the clinician's place in any of these moments, how would you respond, and why?

CHAPTER 6
A Time to Follow and a Time to Lead: Feeling "At-Home" With Circles

Lucia Lopez-Plunkett and Leena Banerjee Brown

Introduction

Carlos is a 2-year-old boy of mixed Latino and Caucasian American ethnic background. His maternal grandparents, an upper-middle-class couple, care for him and his 8-year-old brother. When he was born, he tested positive for methamphetamines, which subsequently led to removal of Carlos from the care of his birth parents. Carlos' social worker referred him for therapy to address his grandmother's concerns, including Carlos' difficulty in "minding" and for "becoming angry easily." Carlos verbalizes very little; he uses grunts and gestures to communicate his needs. The people in his immediate environment are intellectual and communicate well, using extensive vocabularies in Spanish and English. His grandfather is a successful engineer. His grandmother is a retired teacher. Both caregivers are loving and are established in their communities. Carlos becomes lost in his environment, as he becomes easily overstimulated in large groups, is brusque in his movements, and is hypersensitive to textures. Very slight changes in his environment set him off internally and externally, making it difficult for others to understand and connect with him. Therefore, although he is an affectionate, curious, and gentle boy, he is also difficult in his temperament and complicated to understand.

Circle One: "He Chooses Not to Listen!"

In meeting Carlos for the first time, I was struck by his frightened face and intense eyes looking back at me. He appeared sensitive to the stranger in his home and became easily reactive, throwing toys and becoming intrusive in his grandmother's space. Physically, Carlos seemed to be growing well. However, developmentally, he appeared to be a much younger child. The Ages and Stages Questionnaire (Bricker & Squires, 1999) was used, and the results indicated that Carlos fell well below the cutoff score on every subscale except the Gross Motor Scale. First, Carlos exhibited noticeable communication delays, which were evident upon meeting him. During play interactions, Carlos' grandparents often became frustrated with what they described as his nonlistening behaviors. It became obvious, however, that he did not seem to understand what was being asked of him. I asked his grandmother about this, and she disagreed, stating, "No, he chooses not to listen." Carlos scored below the cutoff score in Communication skills, and he scored low on the other domains: Fine Motor skills, Personal–Social (self-help) skills, and Problem-Solving skills. During the course of treatment, it became obvious that Carlos' grandparents had difficulty accepting his delays, and Carlos had difficulty making sense of the (verbal) world around him and coping with its expectations.

Home-based work was set up for its advantage in providing access to the natural environment for assessment and intervention. Carlos had difficulty with separation from his grandmother, his behaviors classically illustrating a boy with a "difficult" temperament (Chess & Thomas, 1996). He demonstrated irregular eating and sleeping patterns, he had a difficult time adapting to new situations and new people, and, as demonstrated during our first session together, he responded aggressively when pushed by his grandmother to play when he was not ready. He was a picky eater: He preferred and depended on familiar foods. Most important, Carlos was slow to accept change; therefore, becoming comfortable in having the clinician, a new person, in his home took a considerable amount of time.

In my first meeting with Carlos and his family, the questions of "What are your concerns with Carlos?" and "How can I help you?" were answered by his grandmother with "I want him to mind." I wondered how aware Carlos' family was about the distinct insults he had faced in his early history and where he was, consequently, in his early social–emotional development. As a clinician, it was important that I obtain the caregivers' baseline understanding of Carlos' difficulties and their beliefs regarding how these difficulties affected their family interactions.

Carlos was born with a positive toxicology report and was separated from his mother at birth because of her drug abuse and her interaction with Carlos' physically abusive father. His mother lived in his grandparent's home while she recovered from her pregnancy; however, she eventually abandoned Carlos when he was 4 months old. Inherent in this information and in the way in which it was given were the possible conflictual relationships between Carlos' mother and grandparents. Further, his grandparents had a limited understanding of the entirety of his insults in utero and their belief that they, solely, had raised Carlos prevented them from understanding that he could have been affected by the separation from his mother. Therefore, they tended to diminish and dismiss both the mother's influence and Carlos' prenatal experience.

Carlos' family is of mixed Latino heritage. His grandmother emigrated from Ecuador, and his grandfather emigrated from Brazil. Although both of Carlos' parents were extremely fluent in English, it was important to his grandparents that he learn to speak Spanish. Because they lived in a suburb outside of Los Angeles, in which the majority of the immigrant families emigrated from Mexico and Central America, finding another family that mirrored the unique cultural makeup of Carlos' family was not easy. Carlos and his brother are of mixed Latino and Caucasian American descent and appear Caucasian American. Their unique cultural background led me to wonder about how Carlos could develop a strong sense of sociocultural identity and how his grandparents could facilitate it (Banerjee, 2000b).

This information sets the stage for *dyadic therapy* with Carlos and his maternal grandmother, a type of therapy in which the focus of the treatment is not necessarily on the child or on the mother, but rather on the interaction and the relationship between the two family members. Carlos was extremely reluctant to meet me, most notably in his grandmother's presence. He became easily overstimulated, grunted at me, and barked out noises while pointing, quite clearly, for me to leave. Despite the fact that I made an initial connection with his grandmother (she appeared open and willing to be included in the therapy), Carlos was anxious about my presence; I was a new person in his world, and as a result, he acted out. His grandmother appeared embarrassed about Carlos' behavior and tried getting him to interact but to no avail. When I asked, "What do you think he is trying to say?" his grandmother answered, "He chooses not to listen."

Circle Two: "I Think the Asthma Medication Makes Him Excited."

The benefits of dyadic therapy in working with a child below the age of 3 years are well documented (Fraiberg, Adelson, & Shapiro, 1975; Maltese, 2005). A nurturing, collaborative, and enriching relationship provides the means for change (Jones Harden, & Lythcott, 2005), which is critical in the synaptic organization and behavioral expression of biological and environmental influences (Maltese, 2005); increases the possibility of resilience to future exposure of stress; and increases the coregulation of calm and sustained interest (Sroufe, 1994).

However, I sensed a resistance from Carlos and his grandmother in engaging in dyadic therapy. In my initial conversation with Carlos' grandmother, I noticed that she had a difficult time maintaining a focus in working with Carlos and wanted to keep things at a social level: For example, she would say, "Your hair is beautiful!" or "What color lipstick do you wear?" She asked many questions about my current pregnancy and wanted to know about my family life. Setting boundaries with her was difficult. She was a determined woman who was accustomed to having her way, and, at times, interacting with her led me to question my focus. On the other hand, my description of Carlos, his development, his language delay, and how his difficulties appeared to affect the family were met with understanding from his grandmother. The grandmother's cues suggested to me that the pace of the therapy should be slow. Therefore, I gently refocused her attention on Carlos' developmental delays and externalizing behaviors. Taking a slow approach, meeting the grandmother at her place of receptivity, and using the grandmother as a valuable informational guide helped me to gently redirect and restructure the flow in the therapy.

Given the level of resistance in the dyad, the approach that I took to deepen the connection between Carlos and his caregiver was to start with providing basic information about Carlos' prenatal insults, his difficulties with self-regulation, his developmental delays, and the services that he could attain to get the most immediate help. Introducing Carlos' delays in development helped Carlos' grandparents understand what Carlos was able to comprehend and respond to in his environment. For example, during an initial session, it was obvious that Carlos did not understand what his caregiver was trying to say; he quickly became frustrated, threw a crayon, and stomped out of the room, screaming. When I commented that Carlos did not appear to understand the grandmother's directives, she indicated, "Oh, he does!" In discussing his developmental delays in more detail, Carlos' grandmother began to understand that Carlos was functioning at a level closer to that of a 15-month-old than that of a 25-month-old.

In explaining that Carlos needed services that would address his developmental delays, his grandmother appeared to understand that his difficulties involved more than what she once knew. She followed through with the referral and began to research his specific difficulties. However, in her zest to find out more information, she began to think that Carlos suffered from autism. After discussing the similarities and differences between a pervasive developmental disorder and the types of difficulties inherent in a child with a regulatory disorder, Carlos' grandmother began to understand that his behavioral difficulties were rather complex and were not characteristic of a child with autism. To begin, Carlos was a sensitive child, internally. He suffered from asthma, was prone to allergies, and often went to the doctor because of recurrent upper-respiratory infections. Although Carlos reacted sensitively to loud sounds and large crowds, he often sought interactions that were of a high intensity. He often reacted in an aggressive manner and became easily excitable when too much attention was focused on him. In describing his sensitive nature, Carlos's grandmother began to gain a deeper understanding of how Carlos' internal and external worlds affected him. Therefore, accepting early developmental services was something that the family embraced for the benefit of Carlos' ongoing growth.

Carlos' maternal grandparents were the only caregivers he knew: His father was absent, his mother's visits were unpredictable, and his primary attachment was to his grandmother. Upon first observation, Carlos appeared clingy and intrusive with his grandmother. It seemed difficult for him to establish trust with strangers and, most important, with me. In the first few sessions, I focused my attention on listening and obtaining enough background history in order to then help his grandmother understand how his early developmental insults affected Carlos. Carlos had a limited ability to establish trust. This distrust alerted me to focus my attention on two important issues: (a) the disruption in his attachment with his mother and (b) its possible effect on his current relationship with his grandmother. My first few attempts at conversation regarding Carlos' relationship with his mother were met with a bit of resistance, as Carlos' grandmother reported that he did not really have a relationship with her. At the same time, his relationship with his grandmother was anxious: He was clingy with her; he followed her when she left the room; and, when others approached either of them, he would move even closer to her by jumping onto her lap. After following her into the other room when he realized that she had abruptly left, he would then have difficulty continuing in an activity because of the interruption.

These observations led to a host of questions. For example, why was it so difficult for Carlos to establish trust? Why was Carlos so fearful of the outside world? And, most important, what are the barriers that are preventing Carlos from establishing a sense of security? In my early work with Carlos and his grandmother, I often sensed the resistance in working too deeply on an issue. The grandmother's resistance and social nature alerted me that she was not ready to face her own relationship with Carlos. The unique dance between Carlos and his grandmother was confusing, intrusive, and unpredictable but was not necessarily harsh in any way. I wondered how much this dance mirrored that between the grandmother and her daughter (Carlos' mother) as well as that between the grandmother and her own mother/primary caregiver.

Overall, the *dance*, or engagement between the two, appeared more at odds with one another rather than a good fit. Carlos' high need for activity was at odds with the grandmother's relaxed and social nature and with her being an older "mother." She often complained that she found it difficult to engage in social activities with her friends for fear of Carlos acting out. Many times, she appeared to ask him to follow her pace rather than engage with him, where he needed her. Daniel Siegal (1999) describes this behavior as that of parents who are preoccupied in their responses to an ambivalently attached child, a preoccupation fed by the parent's unresolved, past issues. The grandmother exhibited a typical pattern in deflecting the difficulties inherent in her relationship with Carlos and in establishing trust with me by triangulating another member of her family.

Videotaping the sessions helped to establish a baseline of the dyadic relationship and to facilitate processing between the caregiver and me in these challenging situations. During one specific videotaped session, Carlos and his grandmother were sitting together, drawing on separate pieces of paper. Initially, the interaction was positive, and the mood was light and happy. Then, the grandmother, a retired teacher, took the opportunity to help Carlos draw sticks and letters with a crayon. Once this change in the tone of the interaction occurred, Carlos immediately became aggressive, scribbled roughly and anxiously, and, eventually, threw the crayons across the room in a fit of frustration. He screamed at his grandmother as he ran out of the room. In reviewing the tape, grandmother explained, "He wants to do things his way." Rather than focus on the grandmother's reflection of herself in Carlos, I took the opportunity to highlight Carlos' developmental level. In noticing the grandmother's frustration and anger in how the session turned, I chose my words carefully, so as not to blame her and to maintain her trust.

I asked questions regarding her perceptions of Carlos' ability to understand verbal concepts such as instructions about how to draw "straight" and "in a row." I reminded her that Carlos exhibited speech and language delays and that much of his developmental milestones were delayed. In the same breath, I praised her for wanting him to do well in school and for trying to help him learn the most basic of drawing skills. I also asked her if she was aware that Carlos appears to understand and communicate through actions and not through symbols such as language. Upon hearing this observation, she threw up her hands and stated, "Then what do I do?"

Noticing her growing frustration in Carlos' behavioral outbursts, I empathized with the grandmother and normalized her frustration. I asked her if I could have "a shot" in trying to connect with Carlos and wondered, aloud, if we could try to communicate with him in the way that he communicates with us. Therefore, I waited until he was ready, redirected him back to the drawing table, and observed him drawing on the paper. I asked him, only once, using soft words and gentle movements, if I could borrow a crayon. This question was met with a strong "NO" and with grunts as a way of maintaining distance. Nevertheless, he invited me in nonverbally by cautiously making space for me at the table. I began to mimic his scribbles, using his same pace and his same level of pressure on the table. He reluctantly responded. In this nonverbal game of connection, Carlos allowed me to bond with him because I was following his lead and was communicating with him on his level. The activity began with a few simple marks and grew into a game of hide-and-seek on the paper, with Carlos eager to see where he could lead me next. As the activity progressed, I changed the object of the game and, nonverbally, asked Carlos if he could then take the next step and follow my lead. Surprisingly, he followed me with delight.

This simple activity set the stage for the goal in relating with Carlos. What was most surprising was that the message was communicated to the grandmother quite clearly, without my having to say, "You don't follow him at his level!" She was able to see it and infer it on her own. Without asking me, she was able to verbalize what he was doing. What was even more remarkable was that she responded curiously and with interest. Therefore, the focus in working with Carlos and his grandmother began to redirect itself, with the grandmother becoming more aware of how to relate to him through actions, thus increasing a sense of connection and communicating "understanding."

Circle Three: "But I Am Calm!"

It became quite clear that the unresolved, underlying conflict in the family easily overstimulated Carlos and many times, he began to voice the familial turbulence. A typical exchange followed in such a way: Carlos' grandmother would ask him to do something, an instruction that appeared easy for a boy of his age to follow; however, when he refused or ignored her, she would ask four or five more times in a desperate fashion and then she would give him an ultimatum. In describing her frustration to me, she would often become anxious, throw up her hands, and give up. This exchange happened often, leaving Carlos angry and frustrated and leaving his grandmother feeling upset and helpless to change the situation. Notably, this power struggle characterized the grandmother's relationships with others in her life, as well. Through his acting out, Carlos voiced an anxiety: "Through all this stress, who will take care of me?"

In helping Carlos' grandmother understand how quickly he became overstimulated, I used her own experience as an example. She often commented about her level of stress, her health history, and her difficulties in her marriage. Naturally, when increased stress was present in the home environment, there were increased reports of acting-out behavior in Carlos. Therefore, the caregivers' awareness of this process was crucial in helping stabilize the home environment. In my growing connection with the grandmother, the means of increasing her understanding of Carlos' experience was to help her focus on her own internal experience.

However, helping her become aware of how her illness, depressive symptoms, and difficulties in her interpersonal relationships affected her relationship with Carlos was not an easy task. In fact, addressing her relationship with Carlos brought up anxiety and resistance; in these conversations, she would often deny that she became angry, carried tension, or had any difficulties at all. This denial made me change the tone and depth of the therapy; waiting for the right timing in which to address these deeper issues was key.

Circle Four: "If the Family Had a Voice, What Would It Say?"

During one phone conversation, Carlos' grandmother mentioned the vast changes in her life in being Carlos' caregiver. However, she didn't elaborate on the changes but focused on the importance of having Carlos and his brother in her care and not in the system. Her situation was difficult. She could not verbalize the big challenge of having to relearn everything in her role as a "mother" rather than a "grandmother." My guess was that if she could have described it in words, she may have articulated "disappointment," as the retirement for which she had been preparing sounded more carefree and travel based than her current situation. She could not address her difficulty in connecting with her own daughter or express her feelings about their strained relationship. She could not admit that the pressure of being a new parent affected her marriage and her health daily. She could not admit that, at the age of 60, taking care of two special-needs children was rather overwhelming most of the time. However, this ongoing instability was something that Carlos acted out daily. He sensed the chaos; he physically vibrated every time the levels of anxiety and tension were raised beyond a minimum in his home.

I wanted to know the strengths and resiliencies that were present and available to the grandmother in her relationships at home, especially between her and her spouse. I wanted to assess the quality of the spousal relationship and the boundaries in their current parenting roles. I wanted to know the sequences of interaction between the spouses around various routine caregiving behaviors. I wanted to know how both grandparents had entered into their parenting roles, how each of them viewed it currently, and what each of their goals were with respect to it. I wanted to know each of their hopes for Carlos as a young family member of mixed heritage and how they wanted to invest in meeting him where he was at and facilitating his development. I wanted to explore with them where Carlos fit and functioned in a structural family map. I wanted to work together with his grandparents to set goals for any desired, realistic changes not only in his developmental milestones but also in his ongoing functioning in relationships with peers and parental figures. These tasks would be some next steps in my work.

Circle Five: "Can You Be My Other Grandson's Therapist?"

When I began working with Carlos and his family, I don't think I was aware of how much this case would push my emotional buttons. In fact, at the beginning of my psychology training, I was not aware of how much I would need to delve into my own personal life to do my job well. From the beginning, I viewed work in the home-based setting as not really "work" at all. It entailed driving to people's homes, being able to make my own schedule, and using play as the primary means of communication. In fact, I often thought that this type of work appeared quite easy, although I learned that it was, in fact, quite challenging. In the beginning of my career, my ambition drove me to want to take on all aspects of the family dynamics, head on. In my development as an Early Connections clinician, I have been learning how to modify that ambition and how to develop my clinical instincts surrounding timing and pacing of the work.

It turned out that Carlos' older brother had a therapist, too, who worked through another agency. This therapeutic relationship was nearing termination because the therapist's placement at the agency was ending. In this situation, Carlos' grandmother took it upon herself (without consulting me) to decide that I would work with his brother, and she provided detailed information about me to this other therapist, Jose. Jose went back to his supervisor and described how he had heard about my work and how he had relaxed his search for another therapist who could work with Carlos' brother in hopes that I would take on the role. Jose's supervisor then contacted my supervisor to thank him for taking on one of their clients and asked if we could help them with others who would need therapists. When this news finally reached me, it appeared that I may have been taking on Carlos' brother, as well, in this triangulated way.

My growing connection with Carlos' grandmother made me aware of her tendency to *triangulate*, where a polarized emotional field/triangle is created in which key players detour and deflect unresolved issues by pulling in a third person and, consequently, prevent their own growth and problem resolution. I quickly learned that I was the *good object*—the person in the triangle on whom others focus their positive energy—and that she looked to me for help in providing therapy to her other grandson. Rather than address her frustrations with Jose's departure, she shifted her focus to me and to "fixing" the situation single-handedly. In her frustration in losing what she described as a "good therapist," she mentioned feeling betrayed by him and his mental health clinic. She explained to me that she wanted to work with someone seasoned and that she understood that this person was leaving because he was working with an intern. She aligned with me and, finally asked if I could work with her other grandson. I was not in a position to take on another in-home client. I had a capped caseload that prevented it, and we were at a delicate and important place in working with Carlos, a place in which it was important for me to remain his ally. I was planning to shift from a dyadic focus to a family focus, in time. Had this shift already taken place, my taking on this additional referral may have been more feasible and also more fair to Carlos' brother; however, at this time, I could not offer to fill the needed role, and I told the grandmother so.

In past clinical work, I have been the *bad object*—or that person in a triangle on whom others focus their negative energy—and I have suffered and learned from it, wanting to be neither the good nor the bad object. I have learned, from experience, that I wanted no part of this trap. As a professional,

I wanted to ensure the best interests of both Carlos' brother and Jose. I extricated myself from the emotional triangle by asking Carlos' grandmother to face her frustrations with Jose and his agency directly, as I had no ties to the policies that his agency held. This action enabled Jose to terminate ethically with Carlos' older brother and to find another agency that could focus on the older brother's specific needs.

Being able to reflect on these issues brings me to a place in which I can learn to address my own self-awareness development and to examine how my own issues and history follow me, even in situations in which I do not think that they will. Overall, the results of these reflected-upon actions were positive: In maintaining boundaries for Carlos' sake, I maintained a focus on the importance of his needs and well-being. It was important that Carlos have his own therapist at this time within a complex family dynamic.

Circle Six: "Am I Being Authentic?"

A few peculiarities arose in working with this family. I noticed, quite subtly at first, a feeling in my body whenever I entered the home. Initially, I ignored this sensation in my throat; a tensing that slowly became more obvious as our sessions progressed. However, in reflecting on this experience in our Early Connections reflective supervision group and in my personal group therapy, I was able to use this sensation as a valuable piece of information for my self-awareness development.

Training in family therapy suggests that the personal development of a clinician is vital in that clinician's ability to work effectively with families (Banerjee, 2000a; S. Minuchin,1996), as self-discovery leads to a more balanced and open sense of clarity within oneself, which diminishes distortions in the therapeutic process (P. Minuchin, 1998). My awareness of the effect that the dynamics in Carlos' family had on me led me to a deeper understanding of my own personal fears and how I respond when confronted with these fears. This understanding has allowed me to see my own lack of confidence, at times, in promoting significant change. I noticed how my gut instinct at wanting to push the family to notice their role in Carlos' behavioral difficulties was coming from my own insecurity rather than from their readiness. I also noticed how the tightening in my throat began to voice a fear of connection with the grandmother.

I was reluctant to connect with Carlos' grandmother because of the experience of being triangulated in my previous clinical work and because of her unexamined tendencies to triangulate. It made me question my ability to behave authentically with her. However, in being more present with her, I found myself developing increasing empathy for what she faces every day. I began to see that triangulation was a way of preventing herself from connecting with the caregiving relationship and, perhaps, its intergenerational history (e.g., "I don't want to know how I affect my grandson."). It felt like a survival mechanism that served to protect the family from its own fears and ongoing family conflict.

In my deepening work with infants, children, and their families, I have often wondered about the differences between center-based therapy and the type of "kitchen therapy" I've so grown to love. I have found that the typical 50-minute hour is far from suitable in my in-home work. Many of my clients belong to different cultures and have different values; different and slower (less fast-paced) time orientations; and less rigidly structured, more relationally oriented expectations of professional help. Respecting these values, expectations, and the traditions of each unique family is critical in the development of rapport and trust. It also takes time to get to know and establish working relationships with each family member. It takes time to absorb the richness and subtlety of the family and community context—for example, the way that a mother gently swaddles her baby in a warm blanket prior to getting on the morning bus, demonstrating her attunement and responsivity, or how the affective quality of a family changes once a father arrives home from work. Families, impoverished and wealthy alike, endure struggles and joys, and merely setting foot inside a home can connect an attuned clinician to the family's unique turmoil and strengths. An in-home therapist "sees it all," but it takes a deepening sense of awareness and self-care to maintain a sense of balance that inhibits the urge to "take it all on."

I was once asked by my mentor and supervisor how it is that I "let go" of that which I "hold" for my clients. I was puzzled by her question and quickly thought of something to say, but the truth of the matter was that when faced with challenges in my clinical work, I was disconnected from the process entirely. Therefore, I never truly "held" my clients or contained their feelings appropriately. I learned this when I began to realize and focus on my internal physical process—the tightening in my throat, the difficulty in taking a deep in-breath, and the ongoing dialogue or song in my head whenever I reflected on a session. This realization alerted me to the fact that I, indeed, was defending myself from doing my work with full presence and, moreover, was unaware of it. I was so often in a self-protective fight-or-flight mode that was typically seen in dysregulated, overstimulated babies, and I "held on" to this emotional weight all day. Until I began to notice my internal process, I was a walking sponge.

But awareness is an ongoing process. Becoming more mindful of how my past haunts me is one in which I willingly engage so as to not be driven by it. I have learned that by becoming more aware of my internal world, I am more able to be awake, become more present, and use various methods to release that which I contain for my clients. This knowledge also helps me to allow my clients to do the work for themselves. This ongoing process has allowed me to seek the source of my shame, which had been instilled in me when I was a little girl. As a part of Early Connections' personal self-awareness and reflective supervision group, I have been able to face these past struggles in a safe and protective environment that allows for growth and an increased sense of awareness and consciousness.

What came up for me in my work with Carlos includes a fear of connection and an ambivalence in my own work, which leads to a tendency to overdo and take on uncomfortable things without protest. My fear in being shamed has limited my ability to voice my needs and has affected my self-confidence. I am learning to free myself of its grip through my increasing awareness.

Circle Seven: "Are My Feelings Really That Heavy?"

Self-care is something that I have learned to incorporate in my daily life. I can now listen to the cues in my body and to my own energy, both of which speak volumes. The energy protects me, warns me, and allows me to be more alive and awake to the fearfulness I once endured. In the ongoing practice of releasing this fear, I have been able to become more attuned to my clients and to my own inner child and to connect without fear of being helplessly drawn in. The simple act of being, so naturally seen in babies, is one that I am relearning. The development of self-awareness and taking care of "me" appeared at odds with the work I tried to do every day. William Schafer (2004) so eloquently described the experience of presence in an infant as "pure awareness, void of content, free from all internal commentary, judgment, comparison, fear, or desire" (p. 5). This phrase describes so well the purest sense of being. The spirit of being truly awake—of being present and true to the moment—is one that has taken me time to include into my daily practice. In my development, the simple act of presence is a growing practice of "letting go" and "letting be"—one that has touched every part of my life. It came out of necessity, and it came because my clients taught it to me. I have developed trust in following and not necessarily in leading. This gift has helped me develop an awareness of how my fears, my shame, and my past follow me wherever I go.

What is involved in taking care of oneself? Naturally, taking care of oneself is not necessarily a relaxing experience. It is the courageous task of looking within and being aware of how past familial turmoil affects our daily functioning. This awareness is most critical in our work with infants and young children, as our experiences so often involve working with and being a part of their unique families. For me, this experience was one in which a sense of shame burdened me, even in the most simple of circumstances: in working with a cotherapist, in presenting to a large audience, in speaking to my husband, and in sharing my needs and wants. I carry this emotion, in which ambivalence and reluctance describe my outward behavior and a willingness to please drives my work and presence. Therefore, incorporating a deeper sense of commitment to myself has been a difficult development for me because I once viewed it as a selfish practice. I often used to say, "I have too many things to do to take care of myself." What I was really saying was "I won't take care of myself" to maintain the familiar, if painful, stance of being self-sacrificing and avoiding the difficulties in my personal relationships.

I now use the tension in my body as a thermometer to help me in situations in which I need to take care of myself before I approach a problem. I have learned to incorporate meditation and relaxation as a primary means of providing a sense of clarity and groundedness in my everyday life. I have learned to accept the compliments of others and express more confidently what I see as progress. The process of addressing the needs in my body takes time, provides space for clarity, and nurtures my inner needs. These processes have given me great rewards in providing myself with opportunities to view my clients and my relationships with them with greater confidence, as well. It does not mean that I do not make errors in judgment, but it means that I have a deeper sense of empowerment and more resources in facing difficult issues. It also means that I can step away from an issue and not allow it to haunt or drive me.

I am now more acquainted with the little girl inside of me who is kind, vulnerable, and caring, the little girl who can learn how to voice her needs without fear. She can also learn how to spot others who will criticize, judge, and shame her because she lets them, and she can use her voice to stand up for herself when this experience happens again. She has learned to forgive because holding on to anger paralyzes her. All of this knowledge has come through self-reflection and peer support, and it has infused my clinical work with new confidence, hope, and energy. These qualities demonstrate true growth and a greater capacity for clarity in my work and in my personal life. Ongoing reflection will create more space to respond to the needs of my clients naturally. After all, becoming more attuned and responsive is at the core of multicultural infant–family mental health work.

References

Banerjee, L. (2000a). Self-development practices for professionals: Gems from the family therapy field. *Psychological Foundations: The Journal, 11*(2), 48–54.

Banerjee, L. (2000b). Through a child's eyes: What's in a name and other thoughts on social categorization in America. *The Community Psychologist, 33*(2), 16–18.

Bricker, D., & Squires, J. (1999). *Ages & Stages Questionnaires (ASQ): A parent-completed, child-monitoring system.* Baltimore: Brookes.

Chess, S., & Thomas, A. (1996). *Temperament: Theory and practice.* Philadelphia: Brunner/Mazel.

Fraiberg, S., Adelson, E., & Shapiro, V. (1975). Ghosts in the nursery. *Journal of the American Academy of Child Psychiatry, 14,* 387–421.

Jones Harden, B., & Lythcott, M. (2005). Kitchen therapy and beyond: Mental health services for young children in alternative settings. In K. M. Finello (Ed.), *The handbook of training and practice in infant and preschool mental health* (pp. 256–286). San Francisco: Jossey-Bass.

Maltese, J. (2005). Dyadic therapy with very young children and their primary caregivers. In K. M. Finello (Ed.), *The handbook of training and practice in infant and preschool mental health* (pp. 93–113). San Francisco: Jossey-Bass.

Minuchin, P., Colapinto, J., & Minuchin, S. (1998). *Working with families of the poor.* New York: Guilford Press.

Minuchin, S., Lee, W. Y., & Simon, G. M. (1996). *Mastering family therapy.* New York: Wiley.

Schafer, W. (2004). The infant as reflection of soul: The time before there was a self. *Zero to Three, 24,* 4–8.

Siegal, D. J. (1999). *The developing mind.* New York: Guilford Press.

Sroufe, L. A. (1994). Attachment classification from the perspective of infant–caregiver relationship and infant temperament. *Child Development, 56,* 1–14.

PART III: PROGRAM AND RESEARCH APPLICATIONS

CHAPTER 7

Thriving in the Clinic: Reflections on Early Connections, a Multicultural Infant–Family Community Mental Health Program

Matthew Calkins, Leena Banerjee Brown, and Michael Barraza[1]

Introduction

The following chapter consists of reflections on the birth and first years of life of Early Connections, an infant, toddler, and preschool-aged mental health program, from conception to implementation and onward. Early Connections, itself, is young and growing, a work in progress. Each day, it faces new experiences, new possibilities, and new challenges, and it meets them with responses that characterize multicultural infant–family mental health ideals and practical concerns in the organization and community. Reflections on this experience tell the story, maintaining the integrity of comprehensive, collaborative clinical intervention with infants, toddlers, and their families despite inevitable obstacles. It is hoped that this chapter will be helpful to agencies and program developers who experience, and struggle with, similar challenges.

---

[1] We thank Susan Carlsson Stone and Bienvenidos Children's Center for their abiding support of the Early Connections training and program.

The Early Connections Population: Reflections on Overburdened Families and Overburdened Systems

A majority of the infants, toddlers, preschoolers, and their families who are served by Early Connections are, in some manner, involved in the child welfare system or represent a segment of the population that is faced with the combination of significant stressors and limited resources. A high percentage of referrals for Early Connections arrive from the Department of Child and Family Services (DCFS) or assorted foster family agencies; these referrals include medically fragile and/or drug-exposed children who may additionally have experienced general neglect; emotional, physical, and/or sexual abuse; and transition into foster, kinship, or adoptive care. A smaller portion of the clients served reside with their families of origin, referred within the community by pediatricians and nurse practitioners from the public health department, local Head Start, and Early Head Start schools or by word of mouth. Thus far, the program primarily has served children in the 3- to 5-year age group, although more recently, the numbers of infants and toddlers referred has increased substantially. Currently, the program serves more than 50 children and families per year. The ethnicity of the Early Connections population includes a majority of Latino (55%) and African American (35%) children, in addition to a smaller group of Caucasian American (15%) and Asian American (5%) children.

Working with such a highly vulnerable group of children and families struggling with experiences of poverty, marginalization, and isolation takes a toll on both the clinician and the service delivery system. It has been documented that individual clinicians experience symptoms of compassion fatigue (Figley, 1995), burnout, and vicarious traumatization (Osofsky, 2004), including feelings of hopelessness, loss, and anger accompanied, at times, by a retreat from emotional connection with others and a decline into disempowerment. The symptoms of burnout in an organization can include inefficiency, low morale, decreased sense of community and motivation, isolation from other organizations, disconnection from the purposes of the work, and administrative rigidity. These symptoms represent obstacles that prevent clinicians from continuing the work at hand in a consistent, dedicated manner.

The first step toward the integration of individual and organizational self-care and the development and sustenance of an infant–family mental health program occurs in the introduction of a less traditional service delivery model focused on collaboration and teamwork, organizational flexibility, and specialized training and supervision. Early Connections approaches the child and family through the complex and multifaceted lens of the Circles framework. To support more comprehensive services for identified children, Bienvenidos Children's Center (BCC) and its program managers reevaluated and altered caseload expectations and productivity requirements, established interdisciplinary (clinician–case manager) treatment teams and a training program that included reflective supervision (as opposed to solely liability-focused supervision), and attempted to redefine leadership and organizational management on the basis of guidelines and recommendations set forth in the multicultural infant–family mental health field (Parlakian & Seibel, 2001).

Despite attempts at implementing new structures and approaches, Early Connections and BCC inevitably have struggled to sustain a genuinely collaborative and strengths-based service delivery. This struggle is due, in part, to the presence of long-standing traditions of Western culture; social constructs, including the primacy of the "rugged individual"; and the efficacy of top-down hierarchies. The fact that most funding sources recognize only those diagnostic categories pertaining to the individual is clear evidence of the influence of these traditions. Despite the presence of social myths, no one clinician—or clinic, for that matter—is invested with the power or wisdom to meet all medical or psychological needs of a person (Foucault, 2003). Nobody can do it alone. However, clinicians and social service agencies have an understandable tendency to fall back into the familiar.

One of the great attractions to multicultural infant–family mental health is that it is entirely relationship focused, as indicated in the *DC: 0–3R* (ZERO TO THREE, 2005) Axis II relational diagnosis, and it has the potential to reinvigorate and transform organizations. By BCC's estimates, it has taken more than a year to redefine our workgroup—including administrators and program managers—from a series of individuals working in the same field to a trusting collective, capable of flexibility and deep investment in relationships with clients and with one another. Our guide through the process was not a prescription or a formula but, rather, the children with whom we worked. Attuning ourselves to their relational needs, we became aware of our own needs as individual clinicians, as members of an organization, and as part of a greater community.

A "Good Enough" Provider: The Precursors of Early Connections

The development of any program requires attention to the qualities of the parent organization and its history of work. Since 1986, BCC has worked in an interdisciplinary context with newborns, toddlers, and their families through a variety of programs, including a residential care facility known as the Village, located in Altadena, California, for children newborn to 8 years of age. In addition to a mental health day treatment program, this facility included the Infant Center, a nursery for medically fragile infants referred by DCFS following prenatal exposure to substances or failure to transition to foster care. The Infant Center program involved a high degree of collaboration among nurse practitioners, consulting pediatricians, residential care staff, county social workers, and mental health clinicians. In 2004, upon the county's implementation of policy changes that removed residential care for very young children from the local horizon, the Village facility was closed. In March 2005,

Early Connections began as an attempt to reinvigorate BCC and to continue its legacy of work with the very young.

The culture of the BCC Mental Health Services (MHS) division contributed significantly to the "provisional environment" of Early Connections. A rather young division, BCC MHS has yet to develop an institutionalized identity and welcomes diversity in approaches to mental health. Additionally, this division has a strong clinical—as contrasted to social work—focus, along with a significant sense of community among staff and a strong understanding of the parallel processes that run from administrators to staff, from clinical supervisors to clinicians, and from clinicians to clients. Managing clinics that are spread throughout Los Angeles County, the administrators of BCC MHS—all clinicians in their own right—strongly encourage, and often contribute to, a combination of teamwork and autonomy and are highly invested in the professional development of service line staff. Historically, BCC MHS has provided individual and group opportunities for staff members to process clinical experiences and to develop increased openness to teamwork, including parallel process supervision, didactic and experiential presentations on self-care and burnout risk, and team case consultation. Early Connections, an infant–family mental health program with a focus on training, reflective supervision, and teamwork, could be nurtured and supported within the existing MHS division.

Movement Through Grief to Hope: Using Process and Context to Begin Program Development

An outpatient clinic began operating on the grounds of the Village residential facility shortly after its closure. At this point, BCC–Altadena had no secure referral streams, reliable revenue, or clients. Morale was understandably low, and grief—manifesting itself in role confusion, sadness, fear, and distrust, at times—was a palpable and inevitable aspect of the work culture at its earliest stages. Matthew Calkins (the first author of this chapter) was a program manager, a position created in the wake of the Village's closure. His role included articulating and reflecting on the impact of loss and change upon the organization and the workgroup. On the basis of Worden's grief model (Worden, 2002), the creation of a multicultural infant–family mental health program to serve as a new version of one aspect of the residential program represents a relocation of the deceased entity, which is the final task of grieving and moving on. However, the tasks preceding this point would have to be observed for ensuring successful transformation.

The workgroup held flexible clinical meetings in place of the more structured and businesslike staff meetings, with the intention of working through Worden's (2002) first two tasks of grieving, including acknowledging the reality of loss and processing associated feelings. Additionally, the workgroup engaged in several frank discussions regarding change as well as adjustment to a new work environment and new roles, representing the third task of grieving. Staff members who developed a sense of excitement regarding the potential of multicultural infant–family mental health began to invest in the program by engaging in marketing and outreach activities to the community. After a period of 5 months, referral lines were established with local area Head Start and Early Head Start schools, DCFS, and foster family agencies. Clinicians and case managers experienced an increase in caseloads from zero to half full, resulting in a resurgence of professional self-value. Although the clinical meetings did not tangibly or immediately contribute to revenue, they helped create the cohesive work culture in which staff members could collaboratively process difficult experiences and be ready to take on new challenges at Early Connections. At this point, BCC–Altadena created a foundation of hope that could support efforts at completing the tasks of grieving by relocating what had been lost into a multicultural infant–family mental health program.

The quality of relationships between administrators and service line staff cannot be undervalued as a factor in program development and maintenance. During times of transition and change, the presence of trust in these relationships is especially important and represents the foundation of hope (Erikson, 1963), a quality required for sustaining engagement in multicultural infant–family mental health. Stressful or traumatizing experiences, such as loss and change, can challenge one's sense of trust in the world, in others, and in the self, and these experiences can result in feelings of hopelessness and disempowerment. In addition to trust and hope, the defining gifts that one may find in life—vitality, creativity, and spontaneity (Winnicott, 1982)—are founded on and experienced within relationships and community; therefore, they can be sustained by the community and by collaboration. Program success may, in fact, depend on the presence of administrators who approach service line staff with the spirit of genuine collaboration and with consistent understanding and empathy of the impact of change and professional context.

Renewal: The Birth of Early Connections

Our first step in launching Early Connections as a program was developing a mission statement and programmatic philosophy that represented the heart and soul of the program. To draw energy for the purposes of the mission statement, Matthew Calkins recalled his own experiences during the Because We Care conference organized by Los Angeles Child Guidance Clinic in January 2005. At this conference, former Surgeon General David Satcher spoke articulately and powerfully on the wisdom of developing flexible, evidence-based programs that focus on addressing attachment in the very young. The key themes of the conference included hope, collaboration, and the message that multicultural infant–family mental health professionals, regardless of discipline or orientation, can work together toward a unified goal—securing attachment in the very young. The Early Connections program philosophy and description was written in such a manner that the team, including administrators and clinicians, could return to it for connection, meaning, inspiration, guidance, and hope.

The Early Connections staff members would have to secure genuine participation of clinicians to ensure that the program began thriving. BCC–Altadena included two clinicians and one case manager at the time of Early Connections' inception. Similar to that of many other mental health professionals, their previous experience had been mostly in play and verbal therapies. Multicultural infant–family mental health was a new idea. We engaged the clinicians in a series of discussions around the program mission and philosophy and provided them with basic knowledge regarding multicultural infant–family mental health intervention. In an attempt to secure this genuine level of participation, we consistently highlighted the idea of choice. Although we faced significant pressures to develop a multicultural infant–family mental health program, we felt it was very important that none of the clinicians felt obligated to participate as part of an organizational expectation. Instead, joining Early Connections was articulated as a professional opportunity for those drawn to the vast potential held in working with early attachment.

Professional expectations play a key part in developing any workgroup. We developed a participant contract for interested staff members and outlined the expectations placed on Early Connections clinicians. By signing this contract, clinicians agreed to develop a caseload with a majority of newborn to 5-year-old clients and to attend a weekly 3- to 4-hour training session that would include a significant amount of self-awareness development and parallel/reflective process supervision, both of which would examine the use of the self in psychotherapy. We informed clinicians in an upfront, honest manner that we would ask them to reflect upon countertransference and emotional responses to their clinical work, with an awareness that such self-examination can, at times, feel uncomfortable or painful. We also informed them that they would be working with a range of intense experiences, from the joy and vitality of witnessing a parent and child connect to the loneliness and uncertainty of felt disconnection. EC's clinicians were to begin seeing cases only after making a commitment to training by agreeing to these expectations. Additionally, we determined that the clinic manager would attend supervision and would carry a small caseload to ensure administrative and clinical integration and collaboration.

One of the key points that Dr. Satcher raised at the conference was the presence of social and cultural stigma of mental health services, particularly for the very young. For BCC–Altadena, outreach to the community and to community professionals was crucial not only to establishing referral lines but also to addressing and working through stigma. At the time, BCC–Altadena's sole funding source was

MediCal, which required that staff members maintain strict productivity requirements. Nonetheless, we readjusted our budget to create an intake coordinator role with limited productivity expectations, and we staffed this position with a compassionate professional who was capable of developing relationships in the community and supporting families experiencing anxiety about mental health services. The funding for this position could have been used for administrative or infrastructure costs, but we believed that basic outreach was an essential portion of a community mental health program. The impact of this role cannot be underestimated. It provides a human face and voice for the program and a bridge to mental health services for families and children.

The Early Connections treatment team perceives itself as a home base for families navigating complex legal, educational, and medical systems. Early Connections clinicians endeavor, from the first point of contact, to make connections with all significant members of the child's life. The goal is gathering a supportive network in an inviting, respectful, and empowering fashion—a network that a family may access with greater ease. Through a combination of clinical assessment and targeted case management, Early Connections reaches out to different levels of need in families—from basic to socioemotional needs. Reciprocal lines of communication are formed between Early Connections clinicians and the family as well as between clinicians and other professionals (e.g., county social workers, public health nurses, pediatricians) with the goal of securing a high level of participation in treatment planning.

Early Connections clinicians attended training sessions in both evidence-based and well-established intervention models such as Incredible Years (Reid & Webster-Stratton, 2001) and Interaction Guidance (McDonough, 2004). As a team, Early Connections incorporated such approaches with a focus that supports clinical development and diversity in our workgroup by encouraging clinicians to develop their own professional style and voice. This focus is facilitated through the Circles model, which trains for competence, compassion, and presence in multicultural infant–family clinicians through the integration of necessary knowledge with self-awareness development.[2] During this launching period, the newly formed Early Connections team experienced feelings of excitement intermingled with anxiety and a sense of renewed purpose tempered with uncertainty. It was clear to the group that we faced intriguing challenges, and a sense of potential resonated throughout the clinic.

Foundations: Training and Circles

To support the clinical work set forth in the mission statement of Early Connections, we introduced Circles as a guiding principle for training and supervision. Our vision of Early Connections involved

---

[2] It is important to note that very few graduates of master's- and doctoral-level programs have been exposed to the mental health treatment of infants, toddlers, and preschool-aged children. Typically, infants are studied as part of a developmental course but are rarely perceived as potential clients.

the integration of technical knowledge of child development, attachment dynamics, family systems, and standards of cultural and ethnic diversity with clinician self-awareness; we hoped that this model would guide us toward a more complete use of the self, in which the clinician draws from the whole, encompassing socioemotional, cognitive, psychohistorical, and spiritual elements of the person.[3] We hoped that this model would give clinicians greater access to *presence*, which we define as aliveness and connection in their work with clients, with themselves, and with all aspects of their work and lives. We hoped that this presence would manifest in the quality of empathy and connectedness, timing, tone, demeanor, and bearing through which good information would flow and affect positive clinical outcomes. Technical knowledge, although valuable and necessary, speaks incompletely and in abstractions to the experiencing aspect of the clinician. Clinical work with children and families often draws the clinician in to powerful emotional states. Some of these experiences can result in disorganizing or painful regressions, drawing the clinician back to his or her own childhood. We intended to engage our team on multiple levels of experiencing, feeling, and thinking so that we could build a reservoir of relational knowledge and experience from which to draw in empathic clinical connection.

From the outset, we determined that our training aspirations required a greater time investment than did that of typical supervision, which can range from 1 to 2 hours per week. Instead, we opted to establish 3- to 4-hour weekly training meetings, and, when the clinic could afford it, the BCC administration team decreased productivity expectations slightly for Early Connections clinicians. Of these weekly 3- to 4-hour sessions, 2 hours would consist of reflective group supervision. The group setting seemed particularly useful for several reasons. It provided diversity of experiences and learning opportunities as well as self-regulating features that led to navigating and organically establishing guidelines and roles that, ultimately, support issues of safety, trust, and group tasks. We felt that this "from-the-ground-up" approach would empower the program and its members to form a live, clinical identity. Our supervisor, Leena Banerjee—the author of this book and a clinician who has more than 25 years of experience working with young children and families—would, at times, be able to step into a role of technical expertise, at other times into a role of peer membership, and, at still other times, into a role of reflective process supervision. The same would be true for other group members. We intended to create an environment in which the team members could step into useful, collaborative roles with one another, resulting in an increased sense of competence and an avoidance of the stereotypical—often narcissistically driven—dynamics of the supervisor–supervisee relationship, including idealization and disconnection from realistic appraisal of the self.

---

[3] Spirituality, in this case, represents the personal—as opposed to the social—journey that one takes in regard to values, meaning in the world, and connectedness to others. It often involves such themes as hope, faith, and humility before greater processes. Human development and the growth of the baby seems, to us, to be such a process. Early Connections does not train, per se, in spirituality but acknowledges its ubiquitous presence in the work that we do.

As defined by Rebecca Parlakian (2002), *reflective supervision* is best implemented incrementally rather than vertically and involves the reflection, acceptance, and clinical use of personal reactions and experiences emerging in practice. Before launching this potentially intense aspect of the Early Connections training, we felt it best to first establish a collaborative work environment grounded by the safest aspect of our integrative model—cognitive learning. For 2 months, the group gathered for a weekly seminar to read and discuss literature on child development; attachment; and infant–family mental health diagnosis, assessment, and intervention. Early Connections clinicians attended trainings in the community hosted by the Los Angeles Department of Mental Health and ZERO TO THREE to continue the knowledge-building process. In addition, we developed a large reference library, including journals, books, articles, and other tools that Early Connections clinicians could check out and take home for private study. In this crucial early phase, the workgroup became familiar with one another, with their supervisor, and with the basics of multicultural infant–family mental health. During this period, cases were discussed through supportive supervision. Assessments also were collaboratively conducted by an Early Connections clinician and the group supervisor, along with a preparatory discussion with the whole Early Connections team and a one-way mirror viewing of the discussion and of the subsequent debriefing. These experiences contributed to confidence building in Early Connections clinicians. Throughout this period of time, the group supervisor (also a program consultant) met weekly with the program manager to connect, discuss the group's progress, and continue a dialogue regarding the growth of the program.

Six months after inception, we began receiving a steady stream of referrals from Head Start, and Early Connections clinicians began to populate their caseloads with children under the age of 5 years. Reflective supervision began emerging organically in our workgroup as clinicians encountered impasses in their work. In such situations, our supervisor would display a significant amount of respect for the workgroup by asking permission to "go deeper." Additionally, our supervisor remained highly attuned to the team members' verbal and nonverbal expressions of resistance or hesitation; to maintain a supportive approach, the clinicians were invited, rather than forced or cornered, into depth. In such moments, it would be enough for the clinician to acknowledge resistance or fear and the needs for trust and safety. Additionally, we established live supervision scenarios whenever possible and reflected upon this situation as a team.

After a cohesive, collaborative workgroup had developed, we could begin the more intensive journey into Circles Five (Self-Awareness) and Six (Clinical Presence). Team members rotated each week, presenting personal material through family genograms, sibling constellations, childhood recollections, and dreams in our 3rd hour. Following these presentations, the group was encouraged to respond to and reflect upon what had been shared. It would be safe to say that these presentations required significant courage on the part of all participants. The process provided group members with the opportunity to know more about themselves. It was not uncommon for group members to experience feelings of joy, fear, excitement, shame, and grief through this level of self-examination before a group. Equally powerful were the opportunities for observing group members as they developed their capacities to hold intense emotional material without disconnecting from the presenter. Through this process, the workgroup developed into a reflective team, which has been extraordinarily valuable during reflective supervision; a deeper knowledge of one another has empowered the team members to speak to one another more directly and genuinely regarding their work.

Collaborations: Opportunities for Growth

Throughout the evolution of Early Connections' training model, we invited professionals to visit our group and exchange ideas and knowledge. Essentially, we were open to adding more voices and perspectives to enrich Early Connections. We were fortunate in that individuals volunteered their time to train our staff members in infant massage and family systems. Like-minded colleagues (from Innerkids Foundation and Mindfulness Awareness Research Center, University of California, Los Angeles) came to dialogue with us on mindfulness and meditation as they relate to therapeutic work. Through these open invitations, a relationship developed with a faculty member of Alliant International University (AIU), who soon joined our group as a clinician and a researcher. As a result, a process research component began. The first cycle of the qualitative phase of this research is covered in chapter 8 of this book. Three more cycles of data have been collected, and a quantitative study of treatment outcomes also has begun. To support this research project, the program consultant/supervisor and clinician researcher obtained a seed grant from AIU. Through this research, we are looking to learn about, and contribute new knowledge to, the much-needed area of training research in multicultural infant–family mental health. We also are studying outcomes to hear—in a systematic, proactive, and ongoing way—the needs, expectations, and satisfaction of our clients as well as the effectiveness of our services. This collaboration between AIU and Early Connections will provide additional support, through data entry, software, and analysis, of both qualitative and quantitative information.

Another example of collaboration came when Michael Barraza, Dr. Banerjee's graduate research assistant whom she trained in family systems therapy, took on the challenge of consulting on an Early Connections case. He did this to help the team generate ideas about expanding a treatment plan from dyadic to family therapy. He is the third author of this chapter, and his account follows:

> *I was fortunate enough to be present during a session of Dr. Banerjee's group supervision in Early Connections with several clinicians who were working with different children in the same family. However, the written materials that were made available to me provided information on only one*

of the children in the home because of all the children in the home, he was the only one being considered for permanent placement with this family.

The 70 documents with which I was presented ranged from individual therapy notes, mother and child therapy notes, individualized education plans, and behavioral observation notes from a play therapy session. Justin, as he will be known in this case, is a 3-year-old African American boy who has been in the custody of an African American family since he was 2 days old. The documents indicated that he had witnessed a number of other children come in and out of this family, and he had been using violence to express his feelings in certain circumstances. His mother has also grown closer to him, as evidenced by her increasing attunement to his needs. Nonetheless, the documents provided me with a picture of an overburdened mother and a sensitive child who was attuned to an emotional void that his mother was asking him to fill.

I used a strategic approach to conceptualize this family because it works well with young children and families and because I am most comfortable with this uncomplicated, solution-focused approach. In this approach, the clinician seeks change by implementing a directive and a motivating rationale, making it very clear to all parties whether or not he or she has joined with the family. In taking these steps, the clinician makes it transparent to the family why he or she is asking the family to change a particular behavior and sequence of interactions. This strategy engenders greater trust, which furthers the healing process.

From the written materials made available and from the supervision session that I observed, I formulated the presenting problem as a 3-year-old African American boy who appears to have severe internal body cue dysregulation with marked developmental delays. This means that he does not eat in any discernible pattern and has considerable difficulty sleeping. He has difficulty using and forming sentences that are longer than three or four words, and his vocabulary is noticeably smaller than that of other children his age.

Justin's foster mother is overinvolved in his symptoms. Whenever something is going on with Justin, his foster mother focuses on the issue and invests a great deal of her energy in trying to remedy the situation. This pattern gives the foster mother a familiar, caregiving-based sense of purpose and also serves to anchor Justin within the family.

I prioritized his treatment needs and goals, which included (a) synchronizing Justin's internal body cues, and (b) restructuring his familial relationships to loosen the enmeshment between Justin and his foster mother. How would I, as a clinician, address these needs and goals? First, I must join with the family, which would enable me to experience the focus of the foster mother's energy and attention on

Justin's dysregulation and the foster father's absence in these interactions and in the treatment process. I would identify sequences of action in this energy–attention focus between mother and son. I would ask the following questions: When does problem behavior occur? (It appears several times a day.) Who starts the problem behavior? (The problem starts when the foster mother focuses on Justin's maladies). What results from the problem behavior? How does it end? When does it not happen? I would then reflect on my responses to the sequences. I would wonder aloud about what Justin's symptoms are hiding. (I might wonder, myself, if this problem behavior stems from possible discord between the foster mother and father or from the foster parents' challenge in establishing a secure bond and repairing the attachment injury caused by the Justin's loss of his birth mother when he was at such an early age.) I would proceed to identify the family's strengths, resiliencies, and felt sources of difficulty. One of the foster mother's strengths is her dedication to Justin. She seems to have made a long-term commitment to Justin by seeking to adopt him. A current barrier is the foster father's engagement (or lack thereof) in Justin's life. I would then develop and administer an effective task to address this situation by giving a directive and motivating rationale.

I would dialogue with the parents using a motivating rationale such as "Mom, you have worked extremely hard in providing for Justin. Through much dedication and sacrifice, you have grown incredibly close to him—so much so that you can read many of his needs and moods well. In addition to your support, Justin's developmental need for a father figure requires that his foster father assume a more prominent role in his life. Justin needs to feel the presence of his dad closer to him. I was wondering if I could have assistance from all of you in helping me help regulate Justin. Dad, I wonder if you could pay attention to the various subtle, nearly imperceptible, signals that Justin's body sends out. Could you provide Justin with some type of system that helps regulate him by placing him on an unvarying schedule, through which he can experience regulation?"

I would continue to dialogue with the parents. Specifically, I would talk with the foster father about how he could set up and implement a schedule for Justin, notice Justin's cues, and connect with Justin's foster mother on these issues for dialogue and support. I would dialogue with the foster mother about shifting her energy to supporting her husband's engagement and being an observer and quiet cheerleader for this shift in Justin's life. I would encourage both parents to bring in any challenges for discussion in future therapy sessions.

In this family, I believe that bringing the foster father and Justin together can be challenging but key in stabilizing Justin's place in the family. It would also offer the opportunity for the foster parents to reconnect with one another and free Justin of his duty to occupy his foster mother's attention in the current family structure. Regarding legal and ethical issues in this family system, I felt that the family's commitment to Justin should be reexamined. Specifically, is his foster mother the only member of this family who is committed to him? Cultural issues also need to be examined. Many African Americans have impressed upon me the prominence of family in their culture. Through the personal account of a close friend, I also understand that people who are not blood relatives are, in certain instances, considered family. My friend told me that he ran errands, such as buying groceries and doing odd jobs around the house, for an older woman in his neighborhood. He considered this woman his aunt, but he actually was no blood relation to her. The fact that Justin appears to have two loving parents may be overshadowed by the possibility that he was brought in to fill an empty-nest vacuum in this family when the couple's biological children left home.

I doubt I could put into words just how validating it was to have the clinicians who had direct contact with the family tell me that the situation I grasped through documents was very accurate. The feedback from the training group was that my plan was very good, with one exception: I did not provide the foster mother with something to do while attempting to get Justin closer to his dad because, at first, I had not developed her observational and supportive role in my intervention. It was as though I was wanting to shift the system in an extreme way, similar to pulling the sun out of Justin's universe and expecting that universe to remain stable. Thus, I came to understand that it was necessary and important to provide the foster mother with a task to ensure Justin's security and her cooperation as well as to prevent her from sabotaging my directives with Justin and his father. So, it turns out that from this consultation, I learned something about implementation, too.

The use of the Circles model has had a profound effect on individual team members and on the development of Early Connections. First, the group's evolution parallels the development of the baby as outlined by Erikson (1963) and Mahler, Pine, and Bergman (1975)—at first, negotiating trust and safety, then seeking protection or support when faced with uncertainty and confusion, and, finally, struggling through individuation and autonomy and falling back, at times, into shame, self-doubt, and fear. The capacity that the group has displayed for understanding, articulating, and processing the very real presence of these developmental steps has greatly informed each clinician's understanding of his or her clients' development. Additionally, it has created opportunities for group members to learn more about their clients through personal and group experiences. The program has benefited by developing an identity that is genuine, real, honest, and accepted by each group member, thus reflecting a true "bottom-up" process. Additionally, the flexibility in roles that the group has allowed has truly empowered each clinician to work with and through their own professional identity and to increase their sense of competence when working with vulnerable children in vulnerable families.

Reflections on Leadership

A young program, much like a newborn baby, carries the promises and challenges of potential. For those who take on the caretaking roles—the parent or the program administrators—there exists a sociocultural setup that the parent/leader makes possible to the fulfillment of potential. Specifically, the parent/leader historically has been defined as the most capable member of a group and stands in a position of self-reliance. However, the relationship between infant and parent is one of mutual engagement and mutual experience. The same is true for program leaders. Matthew Calkins reflects on a personal and professional journey toward understanding the benefits of and challenges to mutually engaged leadership.

It is said that the parent, clinician, and organizational leader is most effective when they are present in a position of curiosity, aliveness, and openness to connection. However, the caregiver can become overwhelmed by the combination of real, external expectations; internal strivings and aspirations for success; and uncertainty. In turbulent and changing times, common to any organization, the organizational leader's capacity to remain centered and to process personal experiences of anxiety, fear, and uncertainty is a core element in ensuring that the workplace culture remains equally centered.

Being both a group participant and a clinic manager was, at times, an unclear role for me and for the participants who "reported" to me regularly. Balancing administrative responsibilities—caseload, budgeting, productivity, and personnel issues—with clinical work carried with it some challenges. During the development of Early Connections, I struggled to manage the combination of (a) administrative expectations that we begin treating infants as soon as possible and (b) the organic pace and direction that the program had taken. Although intellectually, I understood the value of the program's growth cycle, I felt compelled, at certain points, to exert pressure on the program and its participants to quicken their pace, to take on more cases, or to "go deeper" in supervision. At certain times, this pressure was beneficial to the program and the participants, but at other times, it created problematic friction within the group and briefly stalled our course. Regular consultation, self-care, and frequent engagement with staff and other administrators are all requirements for maintaining a leadership presence. The times when I acted without consultation often had problematic results and often set me apart from the group. I continue to meet with the program consultant and the director of BCC MHS weekly; often, these meetings result as much in discussing the program as in discussing the manner in which my role as leader may continue to be effective.

Balance: Final Reflections

Through our experiences at Early Connections during the past year, we have found that despite the challenges inherent in community mental health, genuinely collaborative and mutually engaged relationships across the organization have the potential to sustain, inform, and enrich our clinical work. Inevitably, there are obstacles, within and without organizations, to establishing and maintaining such relationships—fiscal insecurity, changes in funding sources, organizational traditions, and personnel issues can, and often do, get in the way of working in a balanced collective. Throughout the many obstacles that we have faced, we have continued our efforts to reconnect with one another as a team and to work deeply on our cases in the Early Connections training meeting.

Currently, each clinician who began the program now carries caseloads with infants and toddlers, providing in-home and clinic-based services. The tone and culture of the group continues to be positive and authentic, and the quality of clinical services appears to have improved significantly. During our development, we expanded, adding three new clinicians to our team. One of these clinicians serves as the program's clinician–coordinator, and another serves as clinician–participant researcher. One of the original Early Connections clinicians now coordinates an intensive, multidisciplinary assessment program that serves infants and toddlers among its clients. Early Connections now has a membership of seven clinicians.

Our program, while still quite young and developing, has been successful thus far because of a few key factors. The group members have engaged in the work in a committed fashion and have taken on all the professional and personal challenges that have come their way during the past year. Our program consultant has consistently engaged the group and BCC's administration, developing a conceptual framework for the training program. Finally, Early Connections continues to receive support from BCC administrators.

We also have found that the Early Connections program—similar to any multicultural infant–family mental health program—requires the presence of multiple funding sources, community support, and active fund-raising. Fiscal instability—a very real problem in nonprofit agencies—can have a crippling impact on a young program. It is our hope that Early Connections will continue to grow as it is growing today and will continue to receive the same degree of support from within and without. Ultimately, we believe that through the use of reflective processes, multicultural infant–family mental health programs have the potential to assist not only in the development of young children and families but also in the development of organizations.

References

Erikson, E. (1963). *Childhood and society.* New York: W. W. Norton.

Figley, C. R. (Ed.). (1995). *Compassion fatigue: Coping with secondary traumatic stress disorder in those who treat the traumatized.* New York: Brunner/Mazel.

Foucault, M. (2003). *The birth of the clinic.* London: Routledge.

Mahler, M., Pine, F., & Bergman, A. (1975). *The psychological birth of the human infant.* New York: Basic Books.

McDonough, S. (2004). Interaction guidance: Promoting and nurturing the caregiving relationship. In A. Sameroff, S. McDonough, & K. Rosenblum (Eds.), *Treating parent–infant relationship problems* (pp. 79–96). New York: Guilford.

Osofsky, J. D. (Ed.). (2004). *Young children and trauma: Intervention and treatment.* New York: Guilford Press.

Parlakian, R. (2002). *Reflective supervision in practice: Stories from the field.* Washington, DC: ZERO TO THREE.

Parlakian, R., & Seibel, N. L. (2001). *Being in charge: Reflective leadership in infant/family programs.* Washington, DC: ZERO TO THREE.

Reid, M. J., & Webster-Stratton, C. (2001). The incredible years parent, teacher, and child intervention: Targeting multiple areas of risk for a young child with pervasive conduct problems using a flexible, manualized treatment program. *Cognitive and Behavioral Practice, 8,* 377–386.

Winnicott, D. W. (1982). *Playing and reality.* London: Routledge.

Worden, J. W. (2002). *Grief therapy and grief counseling: A handbook for the mental health practitioner.* New York: Springer.

ZERO TO THREE. (2005). *Diagnostic classification of mental health and developmental disorders of infancy and early childhood: Revised edition (DC:0–3R).* Washington, DC: Author.

CHAPTER 8

Early Connections Process Research and Circles: Presence in the Training Experience and New Horizons in Research

Rajeswari Natrajan, Leena Banerjee Brown, Tasha Boucher, Matthew Calkins, Lucia Lopez-Plunkett, Brooke Nisen, and Patricia Rosas[1]

Multicultural infant–family mental health is a fast-developing, interdisciplinary field that is moving forward on the momentum created by strong research and clinical evidence for the effectiveness of early intervention (ZERO TO THREE, 2004). Training and program capacity building are occurring nationally; in many states (Onunaku, Gilkerson, & Ahlers, 2006), locally; and, in some instances, internationally (Banerjee, 2006). The multicultural infant–family mental health literature, thus far, has looked at four questions of significance: "What about the baby? What about the parents who care for the baby? What about their early developing relationships and the context for early care? What about the practitioner?" (Weatherston, 2005, p. 4). Training programs have focused on these questions through the development of evidence-based approaches to work with the parent–child dyad, as discussed in Circles One, Two, and Three in chapter 1 of this book. This research initiative begins a new exploration of the fourth question: What about the practitioner/clinician? Clinicians are the frontline individuals or the instruments who carry out this precious work. The objective informa-

---

[1] Rajeswari Natrajan and Leena Banerjee Brown are first and second authors, respectively, and all other authors are coequal third authors of this chapter.

tion (developmental information, observation models, strategies, and interventions) that they use interacts with their subjective experiences, the quality of their relationships with clients, and their therapeutic styles to impact their work. Thus, including the clinicians' subjective experiences in the training paradigm and attending to the clinicians' learning processes adds new and complementary knowledge to the multicultural infant–family mental health training literature that supports clinician training and the quality of services that clinicians provide.

Some of the essential skills for a multicultural infant–family mental health clinician are their ability to be attuned (Stern, 1995) to the needs of the child, to the needs of caregivers, and to the quality of their relationship. *Circles* adds to this list the skills of joining and being attuned to working with (a) family relationships and community systems in which the parental dyad functions, (b) awareness of the sociocultural/socioeconomic/sociopolitical influences that affect parenting practices and quality of relationships, and (c) clinician self-awareness in relating to these influences and relationships. Thus, a key training question arises from the use of *Circles*: How do you train effective multicultural infant–family mental health clinicians who are attuned, aware, present, and comfortable with holding and working with complex, comprehensive information and complex, interrelated relationships? What processes facilitate such training?

Although training and reflective supervision in multicultural infant–family mental health has grown, the question of how to train effective clinicians has not been empirically addressed. Statements about the importance of reflective supervision abound in the literature, but there have been no systematic evaluations of various approaches to supervision and their effectiveness. A need for evaluation and research on the use and implementation of training and reflective supervision in the multicultural infant–family mental health field has been identified (Heffron, 2005). This study is, hence, timely and significant, as its researchers hope to begin addressing this existing knowledge and empirical gap in the field. Conclusions from this study can contribute to best practice recommendations for training as well as reflective supervision in multicultural infant–family mental health.

Research on training is important for ensuring that training is conducted in an effective and thorough manner. Such research can determine the best processes involving whom to train and how to train (Avis & Sprenkle, 1990; Street, 1988) to produce competent clinicians. So, it is valuable for training research to focus on the process of training. Process studies typically look at the complexities of events that occur within an encounter (Hill, 1982), whereas outcome research typically looks at whether the goals of the encounter have been achieved as a result of these processes (Lambert & Hill, 1994). Thus, process and outcome are closely interlinked. Good process can deliver good outcomes, and knowledge of what elements constitute good process—similar to knowledge of what constitutes good observation, practice, or strategy—can contribute to good outcomes and to more complete evidence. Thus, information on multicultural infant–family mental health clinicians' process expands the training paradigm and the definition of evidence base to systematically include elements that are subjective and objective, intrapersonal and interpersonal, content and process.

Process research first originated in the field of counseling around the 1950s (Heppner, Kivlighan, & Wampold, 1999) and was more recently adopted by the field of marriage and family therapy during the 1990s (Pinsof & Wynne, 2000). Empirical research in therapeutic training has concentrated on outcome. There has not been much focus on process research because of methodological issues such as what to study; from whose perspective to study it; and how to collect, code, and analyze the data (Avis & Sprenkle, 1990; Heppner et al., 1999; Street, 1997; Tucker & Pinsof, 1984). The current research will attempt to bridge this gap by focusing on processes occurring within the reflective supervision group. It will track the clinicians' processes of self-awareness development and technical learning and their connection to felt presence and felt competence in their multicultural infant–family mental health practice.

The Circles Training Model

The Circles training framework that is studied in this research process emphasizes integrating technical knowledge with professional self-awareness to enrich therapeutic presence (Banerjee, 2000; Banerjee & Willingham, 1998). Use of self in one's professional work, or the awareness of an embedded self-in-system, has been recognized as an integral aspect of psychotherapy for a long time (Bowen, 1985; S. Minuchin, 1974; S. Minuchin & Fishman, 1981; S. Minuchin, Lee, & Simon, 1996; S. Minuchin & Nichols, 1993; Rogers, 1957; Satir, 1987). Self-awareness development training has been recognized as the basis for foundational training in the Relationship Competency in the training of clinicians (Polite & Bourg, 1991). This competency encompasses the ability of clinicians to establish relationships with clients that facilitate desired change and growth and the accompanying ability to reflect on these relationships so as to increase self-knowledge and knowledge of relationships (Polite & Bourg, 1991). The quality of the therapeutic relationship (measured by displaying warmth, being caring, giving hope, being motivating, being competent, and exercising appropriate boundaries) is critical in effecting positive outcomes in family therapy (Patterson, Williams, Grauf-Grounds, & Chamow, 1998). The self of the clinician strongly affects this relationship quality (McConnaughy, 1987), and, indeed, the self is the most unique and most powerful resource that a clinician brings to the therapy room, regardless of theoretical orientation (Banerjee & Willingham, 1998). The less well understood the self is, the more it can invisibly distort the therapeutic relationship (P. Minuchin, Colapinto, & Minuchin, 1998), especially in complex relational systems such as a family (Banerjee, 2000).

The Circles training framework emphasizes the importance of clinicians' self-awareness development as well as awareness of their contextual self as it is reflected in their personal family histories, their sociocultural/sociopolitical histories, and how these elements interact with client systems. Such contextual awareness is believed to help clinicians have more personal authority and autonomy in decision making (Boszormenyi-Nagy & Krasner, 1986; Williamson, 1981) and more positive impact on the development of their therapeutic relationships with clients. This can happen through the fostering of a deeper sense of empathy for clients and a clearer appreciation of the complexities of their lives, thus enriching therapeutic presence. In this chapter, we describe the efforts and results of evaluating the process of this intensive clinician training and supervision program.

Setting of the Circles Training

Los Angeles County is actively engaged in building capacity in community mental health programs to provide multicultural infant–family mental health services. Early Connections at Bienvenidos Children's Center is such a program, serving underserved infants, toddlers, preschoolers, and their families. A unique challenge for this program is training clinicians who can do relational therapy that is culturally sensitive and highly attuned to the needs of their infant, toddler, and preschool clients, many of who are preverbal. Early Connections has adopted the Circles training framework that is focused on facilitating and developing clinicians' awareness, felt presence, and competence in multicultural infant–family mental health practice. The Circles framework includes (a) didactic technical training, (b) reflective self-awareness development, and (c) reflective clinical supervision that encourages clinician presence. The framework is interdisciplinary in content and links the fields of human development, multicultural psychology, multicultural infant–family mental health, and family systems therapy. It is within this setting that the research efforts were initiated through collaboration with Rajeswari Natrajan, also a faculty member at Alliant International University, to track and study clinicians' awareness, felt presence, and competence in their clinical work as a result of their training.

Methodology

This study follows a qualitative process research methodology. In conducting this study, we used a significant moments approach to process research (Campbell et al., 2003). This approach has been profitably used by clinician researchers studying child clinical issues at the Tavistock Clinic in the United Kingdom. This framework is based on the belief that learning occurs through clinicians reflecting on their own experiences (Campbell et al., 2003). The research design that we chose to track these significant moments is *phenomenology*, which is a qualitative methodology that looks at the lived experiences of participants and seeks to understand the meaning that they attribute to their experiences (Mertens, 2005).

The design of the study, the data collection process, and the interpretations of the study's findings were all informed by the *constructivist paradigm* (Guba & Lincoln, 1994). This paradigm supposes that realities are constructed and are socially and experientially based. Individual constructions are believed to be known only through active interaction between the researcher and the participants; therefore, subjectivity is an inevitable part of the research process. Ultimately, the findings are co-constructed by both the researcher and the participants, and it is believed that the researchers' personal reflections enhance the contextual understanding of the topic under investigation.

Participants

Seven participants were involved in this study. The training group that served as the participants of this study consists of three clinicians, a clinician–manager, a clinician–program coordinator, a clinician–participant researcher, and a clinical supervisor. The clinicians are all either master's- or doctoral-level practitioners in a mental health field (psychology, social work, counseling, or marriage and family therapy) who are in the process of obtaining licensure. The clinical supervisor is a faculty member of Alliant International University and is a licensed psychologist. The mean age of the participants was 34.71 years (±6.05 years). All of the participants except 1 were women. Two participants identified themselves as Latina, 3 as Caucasian American, 1 as Indian American, and 1 as Asian Indian. Four of the participants were married, and 2 had children of their own in their households. They had an average of 8 years (±7.68) clinical experience. All of the participants reported that their clientele included children who were 0–5 years of age and their families, most of whom were of lower and lower–middle socioeconomic status and attended a community-based multicultural infant–family mental health program.

Members of this training group, who engaged in the weekly training process, initiated this study to begin investigating what they were learning, how they were learning it, and how the training approach was affecting their experiences of presence in multicultural infant–family mental health work. Before undertaking the study, the research was approved by the Institutional Review Board of Alliant International University. Because the study was initiated by the participants themselves and because the research involved studying a commonly accepted supervision process, the study was given an exempt status. However, a consent form (including consent forms for audiotaping and videotaping) was designed for the study, and participants' formal consent was obtained before data collection.

Data Collection

Two methods of data collection were used—journals and focus group interviews. After the self-awareness development and reflective supervision components of their weekly training, group members paused to journal significant moments. For this study, we defined *significant moments* as those that strike a chord, create meaning and linkage to other ideas and experiences, make sense, feel coherent, create insight, and enhance awareness. We requested that each group member spend an additional 10–15 minutes each week expanding on their identified significant moments in their journals. A copy of the journal entries was submitted to the researcher for use in data analysis.

Every 7 weeks, the participant–researcher facilitated a focus group meeting to discuss these reflections. This interview lasted approximately 2–3 hours and was audiotaped and videotaped. The focus group had three parts.

Part I: Significant Moments and Their Connection to Self-Awareness and Experience of Presence in the Room in Clinical Work

In the first part of the focus group, each member got an opportunity to share their significant moments with the group. Participants picked these significant moments from their journals and shared the ones that they considered most important. Following this activity, each member was interviewed. The following questions were asked (Campbell et al., 2003, p. 421):

1. What made you choose this/these as a significant moment(s)?

2. What led up to this/these moment(s)?

3. What followed this/these moment(s)?

4. What did you learn about yourself? How does this influence your therapy/therapeutic presence?

5. What did you learn about yourself as a clinician? How does this influence your therapy/therapeutic presence and competence in multicultural infant mental health work?

Part II: Synthesis of Learning Themes

The second part of the focus group consisted of a group discussion regarding the overall themes that emerged in the individual interviews. All group members identified themes and reflected on the similarities and differences in one another's experiences. The following questions were asked:

6. What themes did the group identify in this discussion?

7. Are these [themes] similar or different from your individual experiences?

Part III: Reflections on the Research Process

The third part of the focus group also consisted of a group discussion. The group members explored whether the process of participating in this research study affected their overall professional development and whether they experienced confidence and competence. The following question was asked:

8. How does the research process (reflections and connections with ourselves and group members) influence each person's development in the field of multicultural infant–family mental health?

Four cycles of data have been collected thus far and were organized by four different self-awareness development exercises undertaken by the participants. These exercises included genograms and sibling constellation; early childhood recollections in familial–cultural context; current and recurrent dreams; and personally–culturally attuned self-care practices. In this chapter, we present an analysis of the first cycle of data from journals and the first round of focus group interviews following the genograms presented in sociocultural context and sibling constellation presentations. The participants reflected on their experiences within their family contexts and the influences of this context on their current multicultural infant–family mental health work.

Establishing Credibility and Authenticity of the Study

The researcher of this study was also a member of the training team who took part in its weekly self-awareness development and reflective supervision activities. The researcher sees clients at Early Connection on a part-time basis and is a faculty member at Alliant International University. In accordance with our constructivist paradigm, the researcher decided to conduct this study as a participant–researcher because of the nature of the program under investigation. The Circles framework used a group format in training therapists and emphasized the importance of integrating subjective and objective information in training multicultural infant–family mental health clinicians. Understanding the group context was extremely important to understanding the group's needs and dynamics. An outside researcher could not hope to holistically understand the roles that each group member played in the organization as a whole and how that organization contributed to group development and change. Besides, in the investigation we aimed to gain an understanding of the process involved in training multicultural infant–family mental health clinicians using the Circles framework and how this process affected their therapeutic presence and competence. Qualitative investigation of these process variables involved being on site and being able to observe the important nuances that occurred during the process of training and reflection (Patton, 2002). Besides, in a qualitative inquiry, the impressions and feelings of the researcher are an important part of the data (Mertens, 2005) necessary in trying to understand a program. By being a participant–researcher, the researcher not only had access to her direct, experiential knowledge of the group process but also had access to her periodic reflections on the process as she participated in all of the different data collection modes. This data was valuable in our attempt to understand and interpret the process involved in the training program.

However, there were some challenges to the establishment of credibility in being a participant–researcher. *Credibility*, in qualitative research, is the correspondence between the way in which the participants construct their reality and the way in which the researcher portrays them (Mertens, 2005). The researcher had to balance participation and observation, ensuring that she could understand the program's processes as an insider but at the same time be able to describe it to outsiders (Patton, 2002). Although this balance was a challenge for the researcher because she was completely immersed in the group process, the interview process was structured by questions that minimized this limitation. During the focus group interview, all of the participants were asked to step back, take a metaposition, and comment on the major themes that came out of the group members' reflections. This process helped the researcher gain some level of objectivity during the data collection process. The researcher also collected data using multiple techniques to ensure credibility. Data was collected from the journals, the focus group interviews, and the researcher's own reflections about the group process.

Another challenge to credibility and authenticity experienced by the participant–researcher was facing the concern that the participants may behave differently when they knew that they were being observed by a person in their group for research purposes. *Authenticity*, according to Mertens (2005), is about whether the researcher has presented differing views fairly and has honored all the voices in the group. The concern that specifically arose in this study was the question of whether or not the researcher should have access to participants' journals. Two potential issues that were acknowledged included (a) participants may not be truthful while recording their significant moments in their journals if they know that their entries will be scrutinized and (b) the researcher must monitor her biases and reactions while reading the journal entries, especially if some of the entries include reactions or perceptions regarding the researcher herself, who was part of the group process. The group discussed issues of safety at the beginning of the research study, especially with regard to the journals being shared with the researcher. The group considered the option of not sharing the journals but, in the end, decided that there was sufficient trust, that they would let their journals be part of the data collected for analysis, and that if a group member's feelings about it changed later, they felt comfortable about bringing it up and reopening the discussion.

While analyzing the data, the researcher had to keep in mind her potential biases and use member checks (Mertens, 2005) to ensure that her interpretation of the data was accurate and authentic. This process involved giving a copy of the research findings and the interpretations to each of the participants and obtaining their feedback. All of the participants read through the research findings and reached consensus that each of them, as participants, had been represented fairly and accurately. As a final measure of establishing credibility, the researcher did a peer debrief with the second author. The original transcripts of the focus group interview and the journals were shared with the second author, who checked for the accuracy of the coding. Some changes were made regarding the coding. Categories were collapsed, and some new quotes were added. Changes were made regarding some interpretations, whereas others were elaborated upon as needed.

Data Analysis

The focus group interviews were transcribed verbatim, and copies of the journal entries were collected. Initial data analysis consisted of becoming familiar with the interviews and with the journal entries. The researcher listened to the audiotapes, transcribed them, and read over the transcripts. The researcher used *axial coding* to further analyze the transcripts and the journal entries. Axial coding is a process by which broad themes, categories, and subcategories are identified, and the relationships between the categories and the subcategories are delineated (Mertens, 2005). The researcher then coded each quote under its appropriate category using open coding, a process where the transcript is read sentence-by-sentence and quotes are labeled according to the themes they represent (Mertens, 2005). She inserted relevant quotes to capture the essence of participants' thoughts. The final step in the data analysis was writing the results. The categories that were coded in the journals were collapsed with those coded in the focus group interviews, when those categories were similar.

Results and Discussion

The results and discussion section has been divided into two broad categories that are not mutually exclusive. They emphasize the different but related foci of process and content in multicultural infant–family mental health training through the use of the Circles model that emerged from this first cycle of research. The categories were broken down as follows:

- How did participants learn?
- What did participants learn?

The first category focuses on the process—that is, how participants engaged in their learning; the second category focuses on the content—that is, what participants learned about therapeutic presence. Subcategories and themes have been identified under each of these two broad categories.

How Did Participants Learn?

Participants had identified significant moments after their self-awareness presentations and after their reflective supervision sessions. The reflections following the self-awareness development hour represented participants' inward journeys of connecting with themselves in the context of their own histories as well as their outward journeys of connecting similarly with peers and with clients. Their focus, however, was on connection with self and with the selves of peers. The reflections following the reflective supervision hours represented (a) outward journeys of connection with clients and with peers focusing on clients' issues and (b) inward journeys of positive momentum, evolving therapeutic style, and personal developmental struggles related to working with clients. The focus in these reflections was on clients and clinical work. Both sets of reflections demonstrated integrative learning processes in which emotional and cognitive processes were actively integrated.

This integrative awareness has been referred to as *differentiation* (Bowen, 1985), or the balancing of the drive and connectivity of emotion with the organization and structure of reason. Differentiation also has been referred to as the dual emotional–intellectual component that facilitates both insight and change (Lieberman, Yalom, & Miles, 1973). Both the self-awareness development and the reflective group supervision activities depended on the group process and on collaboration among the group members for creating a safe, productive, and enriched working environment.

Significant Moments in Self-Awareness Development

Participants identified significant moments in relation to both felt presence and felt competence.

Self-Awareness Development and Its Relationship to Felt Presence

The process of attending to presence put participants in touch with personally experienced barriers to it. Several of the participants identified anxiety and recognition of work yet to do as the causes of such barriers. It seemed that this anxiety was generated by a variety of conditions—for example, wanting to control what is happening, intolerance and impatience with the process, anxiety related to performance/expectations, and so forth. From the participants' narratives, it seemed that the anxiety led to disconnection or cutoff from the process in therapy. Some participants reported trying to overcompensate when they were anxious by doing more than what they needed to do in the interpersonal encounter. Other participants reported that their presence was inhibited by becoming preoccupied with their own issues, reactivity to the ongoing process, and, sometimes, physiological conditions such as fatigue. For many, these awareness came from their own or others' genogram presentations. The group process activated some familiar feelings and dynamics in group members, and some participants were able to identify these dynamics without getting completely absorbed in them.

One participant (29-year-old Hispanic American woman, clinician) reported:

> *For years, I have come to believe that everything I do must be and should be "perfect." In my opinion, there has been no room for failure. I have always been taught to go after what I believe in, but I have also been taught that nothing is ever good enough. In some ways, I have projected these beliefs onto my clients. At times, I find myself pushing them as I have been pushed my whole life.*

Another participant (32-year-old Caucasian American man, clinician–manager) reported:

> *When she [one of the group members, during her genogram presentation] said, "I am done with my father," it [wa]s like a window. I am intent on looking in. I have been told by supervisors that I am often too probing or confrontational. I have little tolerance for obstacles to connection. . . . I get very anxious and uncomfortable . . . when I see like a window for more and this happened with several clients . . . I have trouble with not wanting to open it immediately. In terms of my therapeutic presence, I think that means that I have either cut myself off because I am trying not to be too pushy or I am being too pushy . . . I don't tolerate uncertainty and ambiguity as much as I like. This is something to do with my own difficulty accepting my personal process. Maybe it is a part of me tied up with control and avoiding helplessness. I also wonder if gender plays a part, that is, the authority to know.*

Another participant (36-year-old Caucasian American woman, clinician) reported:

> *Unspoken grief and loss [if not dealt with] make it hard to address [them] in the professional environment. Internalized rage and grief and loss can make you strong to achieve more but powerless in times of distress. [It is] too scary to face the emotions. How to help clients identify [these emotions] and move on if I cannot? [It] is my resistance to want to look at it [emotions] or deal with it. I have a lot of work to do. I am afraid of those feelings. So, how does it influence my therapy? I don't want to go there. I know that I need to, and I know that it is important, and I feel like I will be doing myself and my clients a disservice if I do that, but I find it very uncomfortable and very anxiety provoking.*

Participants reported becoming aware of both the self-awareness activities in which they have already been engaged and of the self-work that they have neglected so far. The participants who reported engaging in self-awareness activities outside of the group seemed to be involved either in some kind of psychotherapeutic work or reported engaging in spiritual, meditative, mindfulness-related activities. The genogram presentations helped some participants identify reasons why they have resisted this kind of work. Participants also reflected on the satisfaction that they experienced from attending to self-work, which enhanced their presence in therapy. The feelings of not being alone and of connecting to self and others were the sources of this satisfaction, and these sources reduced the barriers to feeling present.

The genogram presentations required the group members to be completely present with their colleagues who were presenting and to give genuine feedback at the end of each presentation. This, in and of itself, was an exercise in practicing being present with clients, and the factor that often facilitated presence was the feeling of empathy or connection with the presenter. An acknowledgement that personal processes are isomorphic also contributed to the empathy, the connection, and the feeling of being less alone. Participants also expressed the need for self-care to help them be more therapeutically present.

One participant (33-year-old Hispanic American woman, clinician) reported:

I have been thinking about my presentation all week. Some things came up for me, such as how my past has shaped me and what I have done to not let it drive me. It also shows that this process is ongoing and never ending. In working with clients, I feel like the work [on myself] has allowed me to be more mindful of what issues scares me and what [issues] I tend to avoid unconsciously, which is not in the best interest of the families I serve.

One participant (30-year-old Asian Indian woman, clinician–participant–researcher) reported:

I was so caught up in myself that I was struggling to just be present, and I felt so guilty. When I am anxious, I need to calm myself down . . . I need to center . . . I need to talk about myself. In order to be present, I need to take care of myself first before anything. So, I have been thinking about that a lot. I need to take a moment to reflect and soothe myself and attend to myself. Then I will feel heard and then I can hear someone else and be present.

Yet another participant (33-year-old Hispanic American woman, clinician) commented:

I actually approached the person who presented her genogram. I told her that I felt touched by her openness and authentic presentation. After thinking about this for the past two weeks, I realized it was the entire process that resonated with me. It made me realize that the process of self-awareness is difficult for everyone, as we all have some level of problems or issues in our past.

Participants also reflected on how the self-awareness work has given them insights into, and an appreciation for, what clients do in therapy. Here again, the acknowledgement of the parallel processes in the client system and the therapist system seemed to facilitate presence.

One participant (33-year-old Hispanic American woman, clinician) reported:

So, I guess what I have learned is that . . . that it [self-awareness work] is very hard for me. Being in situations that are so hard for me gives me really an appreciation for what we ask our clients to do when we are with them. They [clients] take this leap, and I think that it takes so much courage and so much strength in a way that I did not realize before.

Another participant (47-year-old Indian American woman, clinical supervisor) commented:

It can be useful to connect with and understand [the feeling of] not [wanting] to let go. This can be especially [useful in understanding] the parallel process with clients . . . if you don't want to let go of a hard past or hard lessons from the past, you can understand when clients don't want to.

Self-Awareness Development and Its Relationship to Felt Competence

Several participants made a connection between realistic expectations of self and the feeling of a general sense of felt competence. A struggle with felt competence was quite evident from the participant's narratives, as well. Insights into this struggle seemed to come from members' own self-awareness presentations and from the group process.

Another participant (29-year-old Hispanic American woman, clinician) reported:

[I have to accept that] I cannot change people and that I cannot control my client or the situations that are occurring in their lives. Part of my personality is that I want to jump in and make everything right, and now I am learning to kind of step back and say that "No, it is OK. Let's see what they do before you want to control and change the situation."

Another participant (36-year-old Caucasian American woman, clinician) reported:

When will I be enough just as I am . . . learning, growing, and BEING? Why am I always looking to some point in the distan[ce] for when it will come together for me and I will feel competent? Why is it so impossible for me to be content with the process and OK with how things are? I think, as I write [this], that I am realizing this is a more global experience for me in my life. Something else, something better, is what I am always striving for, working towards instead of enjoying my life as it is. I am so anxious, hoping for better, fearing for the worst, simultaneously living for and dreading the future.

Participants also gained new insight and information about several issues connected to multicultural infant–family mental health work that contributed to their sense of felt competence. Participants reported that new information, systemic and multicultural thinking, and new awareness of child development and the role of early emotions all contributed to deeper understandings of early development and feelings of competence.

One participant (32-year-old Caucasian American man, clinician manager) reported:

I am reminded of how often I tend to think in nuclear terms . . . in homogenous terms at the expense of cultural difference. The genogram presentations confront me with this. I am reminded of my limited way of articulating one's journey. I am missing a lot, I think. I think I may be too focused on the internal aspects of a person instead of on [the broader aspects]. I need to incorporate [systemic thinking]. It is like a relief, sometimes, to see that there is so much more.

Another participant (29-year-old Hispanic American woman, clinician) commented:

I have come to truly see the differences, fears, and worries among various cultures. I especially see this within the Latino community. So many of my clients' parents lack appropriate knowledge and support regarding any and all mental illness. Additionally, they lack reassurance and awareness regarding what is [the] appropriate parenting style and discipline.

Yet another participant (30-year-old Asian Indian woman, clinician–participant researcher) reported:

I was struck by the vivid images [memories] that she [one of the group members] had as a child, in her mother's lap watching her baby brother being buried. What can a child understand? She obviously knew [even as such a young child] that something was wrong, and that image stuck to her mind. How powerful!

Another participant (32-year-old Caucasian American man, clinician manager) reported:

Rage or anger appears common in families, [and it is] particularly active in early childhood and adolescence. As of now, it appears to serve a similar purpose for each [person who shared their genogram] . . . the need to put a voice to an unpleasant, unheard experience.

Discussion of Self-Awareness Development and Its Relationship to Presence and Felt Competence

Presence has been defined as being totally in the moment—in body, mind, and emotions (Geller, 2001). *Circles* consolidates this definition and those presented by Bugental (1978), Csikszentmihalyi (1990), and Siegal (1999) to define *presence* in the following way:

That feeling of aliveness and connection with an infant and her family in which the clinician is fully absorbed and engaged and feels access to her own experiences and those of her clients with enjoyment, vitality, and informed awareness, being centered and in sync in the moment.

Nonpresence occurs when the clinician enters the session with a particular agenda or a preconceived notion of what needs to be worked on and does not allow space or openness for the client's own agenda to emerge (Geller, 2001). Anxiety results from this *dissonance*, or incongruence between the clinician and the client (Rogers, 1957). Excessive anxiety or holding in the relationship leads to disconnection (Sameroff & Mackenzie, 2003). Expressions of this anxiety clearly come through in the narratives of the study participants and seem to hinder their therapeutic presence.

Self-awareness and self-development have been implicated in building this capacity for presence (Keefe, 1975; Lietaer, 1993). According to Kempler (1970) and Webster (1998, as cited in Geller, 2001), a clinician has to be psychologically well developed and integrated, with insight and access to his or her own self and vulnerabilities. A clinician cannot be open to a client's experiences if he is not open to his own experiences (Lietaer, 1993). It has been stated that clinicians who are not self-aware may tend to minimize problems and issues that clients bring in and also may set themselves up for superficial therapeutic relationships (Timm & Blow, 1999). According to Hycner and Jacobs (1995), a clinician who has not paid attention to her own pain and level of injury is often preoccupied with herself and does not have enough room for being in touch with injured and disowned parts of clients. The literature also points out that clinicians who focus on the client system to manage their anxieties will end up being controlled by the ups and downs of this system, whereas clinicians who focus on self to manage anxiety will be more grounded and balanced while working within an unstable client system (Schur, 2002). Bowen's (1985) differentiation model, which provides intrapersonal and interpersonal pathways for self-awareness development, is similarly anchored in self. Clinicians in Early Connections reflected on connecting with themselves as well as seeing themselves as not alone in their pain as ways of reducing barriers to presence.

One method of working with self-awareness development is the use of *genograms*, or family diagrams of the family of origin. According to Bowen (1985), going back to family-of-origin issues and working through them helps clinicians work from a nonreactive and nonanxious place, regardless of what is being presented in the therapy room. From this position, the clinician can attempt to use his emotional reactions to inform his work rather than distract him from it. Literature also supports the view that clinicians who experience self-awareness development work have greater respect and empathy for the struggles of their clients (McDaniel & Landau-Stanton, 1991).

Three stages have been delineated in the process of developing therapeutic presence (Geller, 2001): (a) preparation, (b) process, and (c) the experience of presence itself. In the preparation phase, clinicians enhance their opportunity for presence, and one way to do this is by working on one's self-awareness development issues. It appears that participants of this study are well into the preparation phase because they clearly have developed an awareness of the need for self work and an awareness of their common patterns and dynamics of engagement.

As an individual begins to verbalize and use language to access and understand her own life experiences, she begins to coordinate neurological systems (Deacon, 1997) and build a coherent and integrated sense of self (Maturana & Varela, 1987), which is crucial in the development of presence (Kempler, 1970). The Early Connections group also is demonstrating the second stage by beginning to integrate emotional and cognitive awareness gained through intrapersonal and interpersonal connection. The experience of connection itself is occurring, at times, in described moments of attuned therapeutic connection as well as experienced movement and change in clients. For a young group of multicultural infant–family mental health clinicians, this appears to be a realistic and authentic pace of movement.

The process of self-awareness development work also has been cited as a medium through which discourses regarding race, ethnicity, class, and gender can be held and through which therapists can be made sensitive to these contextual issues (Lawless, Gale, & Bacigalupe, 2001). According to the authors, such activities subtly bring these contextual variables into the supervisory dialogues, which may be more effective than formally introducing these topics for analysis and discussion. It seemed that even the cognitive understanding of issues such as child development were enhanced by the study group's self-awareness development activity. McDaniel and Landau-Stanton (1991) state that personal experience with the material may provide a very different kind of learning that deepens the understanding that emerged when the same material was taught in the conventional way.

Group Process Variables

From the participants' narratives, it appeared that several specific group process elements may have contributed to the participants' insights about therapeutic presence and felt competence. It is important that we comment on these group process variables because they may help in understanding what processes contribute to generating and sustaining reflection and self-awareness.

Several participants identified the aspect of gaining trust as an important variable in helping them engage in the process of self-reflection. Some participants reported feeling apprehensive about doing self-awareness work in the group. Others reported that seeing others do the work and finding commonalities in their presentations helped them gain trust and feel confident about doing the work themselves. The perception of the group being a cohesive, safe unit was noted as something that helped participants gain trust.

One participant (36-year-old Caucasian American woman, clinician) reported:

> *I never thought that we all could have had so much [in common]. I connected with people just from their presentation at such a different level and . . . I felt so much emotion when everybody was presenting. I was very surprised by that. I think that, ultimately, for me [this process] has helped to gain more trust and be more open than I do think [I would have been].*

Another participant (33-year-old Hispanic American woman, clinician) reported:

This [the genogram presentation] is really a thorough process, and I was very scared. I guess I do not talk about my family to really anyone. I was wondering how safe it will be for me to share my family genogram. The group seemed cohesive, and there was an air of safety where touchy subjects could be discussed freely.

Another aspect of the group process that seemed to help participants in their self-awareness work was getting feedback from other participants about their presentations. It seemed that the group members were like mirrors that participants used to reflect on themselves and to gain a better sense of self.

One participant (29-year-old Hispanic American woman, clinician) reported:

It made me realize that we have a lot of similarities amongst each other, and so it does not make me feel like I am different. I feel like I am part of everyone's life here. In each of their genograms, there was a little part of me. [I was able to recognize myself or sometimes realize that] this is what I want. Just hearing them made me see what I can change because it is possible to change that part.

Another participant (36-year-old Caucasian American woman, clinician) reported:

I hadn't yet incorporated feelings of anger towards my mom and [decided] how to depict it in my genogram. It is almost like her [one of the group member's] discussion about her mother gave me permission because now I do feel like I could discuss anger towards my mom for her choices. The last thing I took away from the [genogram] experience and the most powerful was the group's feedback about resilience. I am still reeling as this is not my general experience of myself. I always see where I haven't measured up to my own expectations and how my experience of being raised and to some extent raising myself only hurt me and that things could have been so much better for me if only that stuff hadn't been my reality. Resilience, however is a much better place to live and I will try.

Another participant (30-year-old Asian Indian woman, clinician–participant researcher) reported:

Everybody punctuated something about me or my relationships while giving me feedback. I still remember the feedback about how [my presentation] was poignant and about the connection that I have with my mom. I hold on to it [the feedback] because it punctuated something for me, and what a nice gift it is [for me] to see it. I initially thought that I was not going to get anything out of it.

Several participants also seemed to agree that making self-awareness development work a discipline or a routine process in one's mainstream therapeutic work was important. The participants implied that the group setting was conducive in making a commitment to that self-awareness development work.

One participant (47-year-old Indian American woman, clinical supervisor) commented:

> *I do think [of] being in this group as having a regular place to commit to explore [one's own self] and to journey together. It has done something for me in terms of opening the door for [exploring some early feelings and recollections]. [Those experiences] are already wordless, and it is very easy to put [them] away and keep [them] locked up . . . but [to have the opportunity to explore them] in the mainstream of one's work is a powerful tool.*

Discussion About Group Process Variables in Self-Awareness Development

The process of building trust and safety in a group is a normal process and is especially important when therapists are getting ready to work on their family-of-origin issues (Thistle, 1981). It seems that the feeling of apprehension is common, as most therapists think that their "family's brand of pathology is unique" (Thistle, 1981, p. 250), but once they see similarities in other families, feelings of trust and safety follow. This experience allows the therapists to open up and be more introspective (Thistle, 1981).

As Yalom (1995) has stated, a freely interactive group, given time, develops into a social microcosm of the participant members. Here, the group members begin to play out their characteristic dynamics. Sometimes, group members act as mirrors to others in the group, thus helping one another reflect on aspects of their selves. Similar to two mirrors facing one another, each group member provides a self-consistent reference for the other (Wolf, 1988). Thus, participants can use the group as a laboratory to gain clarity and meaning behind their dynamics and behaviors. However, before this can happen, the group members must be able to cognitively process and reflect on their emotional responses. Literature shows that the strong emotional experience, alone, is not sufficient and that the dual emotional–intellectual component needs to exist for insight and change to occur (Lieberman et al., 1973). From the participants' narratives, these dual processes are occurring in the Early Connections group.

Significant Moments in Reflective Supervision

The significant moments in the reflective supervision sessions came from the synergistic group discussions that participants held about clinical cases; these discussions focused on felt presence. Participants experienced the group process as greatly facilitative of new learning; of being invigorated, excited, and vulnerable; and of finding voice as clinicians. Participants reported active engagement with their own development as clinicians.

Role of the Group's Presence in Facilitating Clinicians' Presence and Ability to Achieve Higher Levels of Integrative Learning

The reflective group supervision brought an excellent sense of growth and success to the group and increased their morale. The participants were able to see movement in their cases with the help of the group process, which invigorated them.

One participant (32-year-old Caucasian American man, clinician manager) reported:

> [I]really felt alive in a moment of shared experience [about the] grief and loss regarding the two patients. It felt enormous, palpable, and so real. It felt alive, and the group digested that which the mother [the client's mother] cannot.

Participants were able to reflect on their countertransference issues as these issues related to their clinical process. This process reflected the integration between the learning that participants gained in their self-awareness work and their clinical experience.

One participant (36-year-old Caucasian American woman, clinician) reported:

> The anger [that was part of the counter transference] was propelled into understanding and awareness by processing in the group. New insight to move . . . to grow and [to regain] positiveness.

Another participant (36-year-old Caucasian American woman, clinician) shared:

> I spoke up in the group [regarding a case] and then felt horribly guilty. I spoke up, and it is so wrong. It is so uncomfortable for me to challenge anybody . . . especially in therapy, I really have a hard time giving feedback. . . . especially in dyadic therapy. I [worry] that the mom [client's mom] would perceive me as challenging. I think I really have a hard time being the bad object or being perceived as somebody really bad. The thing that makes me sad is that I am just so sorry all the time, so guilty. I know where this comes from, of course—childhood—but it is still with me, weighing me down, and it is tiring. I usually don't give myself permission to show up in any way that is challenging or could be perceived as challenging.

Yet another participant (32-year-old Caucasian American man, clinician–manager) shared:

> This mother [client's mother] is so symbolic. I feel lost and helpless, but I know that, truthfully, rage or great anger is what I feel most. . . . The group helped me see my own dramatic role. Different voices reflecting different parts of that complexity.

Clinicians reported reflections on their emerging therapeutic styles as multicultural infant–family mental health clinicians. They were organizing the lessons learned and meshing them with their characteristic ways of being in, and approaching, therapy. This process reflects an ability to achieve a higher level of integrative learning.

One participant (36-year-old Caucasian American woman, clinician) reported:

How to attempt to make sense of chaos within a system, and how to look at what is presented with intensity and confusion [ambivalence], how to hold and know where the line of abuse lies? Not taking too much on and remembering my role.

Another participant (32-year-old Caucasian American man, clinician–manager) shared:

Identifying with the child is the first step, building rapport and holding the parent is the next . . . the description of attachment as involving consistency and emotional presence clarifies this dynamic considerably. Bringing technical awareness to a parent is one of the best ways to begin to engage.

Yet another participant (36-year-old Caucasian American woman, clinician) shared:

The take away is to slow down and be attentive to the process. This really represents a shift for me and also feels like, perhaps, my natural way of interacting with clients: slowly, with attention, always with the relationship in mind. The next step is for me to really get the experiential aspect of all this, in terms of understanding in the moment, in the session and transfer that information by voicing my understanding in a way that will help the dyad/family.

Discussion About the Role of the Group's Presence in Facilitating Clinician's Presence and Ability to Achieve Higher Levels of Integrative Learning

From a systemic perspective, it is assumed that the reflective group process/system could be part of the system of therapy between the participant and the client. A criterion that indicates whether the reflective group process is working is the presence of movement or momentum in the group members (Schur, 2002). According to Schur (2002), movement with momentum supports a view in which a system is flexible and self-organized without external support for stability. In the participants' narrative, evidence of this momentum is "manifested as excitement as well as vulnerability about the changes and about the understanding of the systemic patterns" (Schur, 2002, p. 413) in the client, therapist, and supervisory systems.

Participants' reflections in the journals and in the focus groups demonstrated integrative learning processes in which emotional and cognitive processes were being actively integrated. Because the self-awareness development hour preceded the reflective supervision hour, the seeds of trust, safety, and integrative learning that were sown after this hour were further integrated into the reflections following the reflective supervision. This higher level of integration meant that participants were beginning to articulate issues of personal clinical style, strengths, and needs in their discussion of self in the context of their multicultural infant–family clinical work.

What Did Participants Learn? Themes Regarding Therapeutic Presence

Several themes were identified that reflected different aspects of therapeutic presence in multicultural infant–family mental health. These themes were especially emphasized in the focus group interview.

Being and Doing

It seemed that the participants were engaged in understanding the meaning of the terms *being* and *doing* and their connection to therapeutic presence. The differences between the two were processed, and the participants seemed to agree that being was strongly associated with therapeutic presence. *Anxiety* was identified as something that interferes with the state of being, and participants discussed ways of achieving this state. Most participants seemed to agree that doing was easier than being in a state of being, with the latter requiring a lot of practice. However, the participants also acknowledged the paradox that in being with your client, you are activating the process of therapy that seems as though you are doing something therapeutic with your clients. Being also was equated with the acts of holding and containing. Participants spoke of the nature of the therapeutic work with infants who are preverbal as being very different from the work with adults, who are verbal. The changes facilitated in multicultural infant–family work can be more subtle than in therapy with adults only. The therapist was thought of as a crucible who could hold the clients, undisturbed, as they worked through their issues; the clinical supervisor was thought of as a crucible who could hold clinicians in reflective supervision in a similar way. In the end, the participants concluded that a balance between the two states of being and doing was necessary in order for the self to be truly regulated and present.

One participant (33-year-old Hispanic American woman, clinician–coordinator) commented:

> *Maybe, from outside, it looks like nothing happened [in therapy], but the truth is that we are doing much more than what appears [on the outside]. I am tolerating . . . I am holding . . . I am saying that it is "OK." [It is sometimes] an exchange that happens internally with the client and with you. That has such a profound impact, and, I think, in all of our lives, not just [those of] the clients.*

One participant (33-year-old Caucasian American man, clinician–manager) reported:

> *You [the clinical supervisor] made the comment about a paradox, that in order to move and to change, you need to hold. It is a paradox because . . . it goes to this "being versus doing" thing, and to change, you have to be still and settled, and that really come[s] into conflict with the part of me that wants to create some change immediately, which I want to do. So, I am just learning more about being still.*

Another participant (47-year-old Indian American woman, clinical supervisor) reported:

> *I am realizing now [that being] has a lot more to do with connecting with those feelings within yourself. . . . within your early self. You must be very comfortable with holding but also be comfortable with becoming a catalyst when that moment arrives, and I think [there needs to be a] balance between [being and doing].*

Yet another participant (36-year-old Caucasian American woman, clinician) shared:

> *I am thinking that if people can approach [being and doing] from that middle place . . . from that place of stillness . . . it means that you can be still even while doing. It is centered, not reactive.*

Attunement and Timing of Intervention

The participants reported that the realization that attunement and timing of intervention were aspects of therapeutic presence was significant. They reported that they learned the necessity of pacing their interventions to fit their multicultural infant–family clients. Another significant lesson that they reported was seeing the meaning and opportunity in the moment for connection through the attunement process. Along with the idea of timing of intervention, the importance of paying attention to and understanding the client's developmental capacities also was noted as a significant learning point.

One participant (30-year-old Asian Indian woman, clinician–participant–researcher) reported:

> *When we were talking about this particular case, we had all these ideas, and my suggestion was to bring in the client and have us all give her feedback. That is when you [clinical supervisor] said that the process of conceptualization is very different from the process of intervention . . . that is, what is important in intervention is timing. I have, ever since then, been thinking about timing in intervention.*

Yet another participant (47-year-old Indian American woman, clinical supervisor) commented:

> *[In multicultural infant–family health work] you are not doing 20 million things. You are doing only a few things that will [in turn] affect the 20 million things. The pace and the entry are different. At a very young age, the capacities to do 20 million things have to be developed.*

Attitude Toward Time and Its Relation to Connection and Regulation

Several participants discussed that a significant learning moment was understanding the relationship between one's attitude toward time and the concepts of connection and regulation. The importance of slowing down and connecting to the idea that time is infinite was acknowledged. This slowing down was related to the ability of connecting to oneself and achieving self-regulation. Participants also shared how this attitude toward time gives them the clarity and direction to create change.

One participant (36-year-old Caucasian American woman, clinician) commented:

During anxiety-provoking moments, [it is important to] slow down and remember to connect to self. Slowing down before I decide what to do helps [me] regulate my own self . . . give clarity and awareness.

Another participant (47-year-old Indian American woman, clinical supervisor) shared:

I found that slowing down and remembering this idea of infinite time gives perspective. It requires an understanding, a real-time experiential connection with the infinite, the eternal nature of things. . . the ongoing ever-changing nature of things. It speaks to me of the importance of stopping, letting in, experiencing, connecting, and savoring the different aspects of what we are doing. You can see yourself, then, in some kind of greater perspective, and so it allows connection to self. [This connection] is telling me about my own experience in the moment. I can slow down and treat that with the respect that it deserves. What I have been finding is that . . . that itself is so key to a deeper level of regulation. How do you regulate with deeper, more respectful connection to self? If I actually stop and let that happen, it fills me, and I know what to do after that. Things flow . . . there is presence.

Yet another participant (30-year-old Asian Indian woman, clinician–participant–researcher) reported:

Even if you have connected for 5 minutes, it seems like infinite time, and we are able to have that clarity and the energy to make a shift.

Discussion of Themes Regarding Therapeutic Presence Generated Through the Reflective Group Supervision

A challenge for those involved in the Circles training is the fact that, unlike other therapeutic skills, therapeutic presence is not a technique that can be taught. It is more fundamental. Presence is something that is needed for techniques to work (May, 1958). Techniques follow naturally from presence, the latter coming from commitment and time given to becoming one with self and with one's surroundings (Geller, 2001). Geller (2001) says that the act of committed and regular self-exploration, identified as a significant theme by the participants in this study, leads to activating forces that generate presence. The themes recognized from the reflective group supervision seem to point to the attitudes and the ways of being that are necessary for activating these forces.

The first theme regarding being and doing has been recorded in literature as an important aspect of having therapeutic presence. Being with a client has been noted as healing in itself (Santorelli, 1999).

Congruent with the ideas that emerged from the participants' narratives, Santorelli (1999) also states that presence involves a quality of nondoing but not inactivity. He adds that from this place of nondoing, appropriate responses and interventions can emerge.

A case has also been made for centeredness, or balance, in literature, which also is an expression of personal integration and a unity of body and mind (Clark, 1979). *Centeredness* is described as a nonreactive position that carries a paradox of detachment and involvement (Clark, 1979). Centeredness is said to be important for a clinician so that he can deeply take in the client's experience (being) and be able to remain calm in the midst of it so as to intervene as needed without being constrained (Hycner, 1953).

Timing is also an important theme that has been talked about in the literature. Prochaska and Prochaska (1999) identify different stages that clients go through in their journey to create changes: precontemplation, contemplation, preparation, action, maintenance, and termination. They note that, sometimes, no matter what techniques or interventions therapists use, clients do not change because they are not yet ready for change to happen. This highlights the importance of timing in interventions, especially a sense of timing that comes from being present and highly attuned to the needs of the client system. As the Zen saying goes, "When the disciple is ready, the teacher arrives," it appears that the multicultural infant–family mental health clinician's task is being closely attuned to the state of receptivity of the client system and intervening when clients are ready to receive.

Another theme identified by the participants as key to therapeutic presence is one's attitude toward time. Rotenstrich (1967) noted that presence involves the suspension of chronological time in which the future and the past dissolve. This attitude of being completely absorbed and connected with another person in the present time seems to carry with it a quality of being in a timeless encounter (Geller, 2001) that can be deeply healing. Even in physical science, it has been theorized that when matter connects or collapses under the gravitational pull to form a high-density medium (such as in black holes), the property of time slows down (Wolfson, 2003). This theory resembles the experience that people have when they connect with self or with one another at a profound and deep level that produces healing outcomes.

Reflections on the Research Process

The process of the research study was not discussed as a theme in the journals. However, during the focus group interview, this theme was explored. The research process involved the activities of journaling, the focus group interview, and member checks, and these activities seem to have functioned as a focusing lens that helped participants bring together, organize, and integrate their learning. This integration of learning seems to have happened through the processes of engaging in personal reflection (journaling), participating in interactive dialogue (focus groups), and reading about the process of their own learning and its content (member checks). The research process was seen as a space in which participants could bring their various pieces of learning under focus, reflect on them, and organize them in a meaningful way that they could then internalize.

One participant (47-year-old Indian American woman, clinical supervisor) reported:

What this research did for me is to identify a moment in there . . . to stop and gather that thing that I wanted to hold on to. I felt that it was a gift to me . . . to take a moment, to experience it, and to let it change me.

Another participant (36-year-old Caucasian American woman, clinician) shared:

After reading the chapter, I felt a deep sense of appreciation for the work we had all done together. I felt proud of our accomplishments as a group and the growth [that] we had all experienced. I also felt as if reading about what we have undertaken as a group thus far really synthesized my experience for me and created a more complete, even linear, understanding of what we have been doing. The whole experience for me, of course, has been experiential thus far, and in that way, reading such a fully fleshed out summary of our work made it all come together for me. It actually fueled a greater sense of excitement for what we are doing. In that sense, reading the chapter made me want to continue to engage with the work with energy and perhaps a little more passion than before.

Conclusion

In going through this journey of self-awareness development, reflective supervision, and the process research on significant moments, what we bring to the multicultural infant–family mental health training platform is our understanding that integrative learning occurs effectively when we engage in this training sequence systematically in a group setting. From a very small subset of our data set, we can see that including the clinician's self-awareness development training systematically before engaging in a case discussion using group processes in which trust, safety, and mirroring were reliably and skillfully established led to progressively integrative learning for clinicians. Such a setting not only enhanced intrapersonal and interpersonal learning and connection but also helped clinicians transfer intrapersonal/interpersonal knowledge from the context of self, family, culture, and peers to the therapeutic context. The group process was a key vehicle that facilitated clinicians' ability to transfer this knowledge from the personal to the professional/therapeutic realm. This experience, ultimately, contributed to felt therapeutic presence and competence and prepared clinicians for the parallel experiential processes with clients. It also transformed Circles from a static conceptual framework to a live process framework in which Circle Five, Self-Awareness Development, catalyzed simultaneous access to intrapersonal and interpersonal information in all of the circles/domains.

Our experience with the research process also brings to bear the fact that seeking evidence for change or development during the training process involves tracking subtle relational processes that occur within the trainees, among the trainees, and between the supervisor and the trainees. These processes are isomorphic to processes in multicultural infant–family mental health work in which the clinician must track subtle processes within the infant, between the caregiver and the infant, and between the clinician and the client system. These processes comprise a complex array of variables, some of which can be observable behaviors and some of which can represent abstract thoughts. The apparent difficulties in quantifying such subtle process variables calls for alternative methodologies that can help us track these variables and provide us with an expanded, richer, more complete evidence base. The qualitative significant moments approach used in this study—specifically, adopting the phenomenological design—lent well to tracking these subtle process variables in the training context. Future research needs to explore further creative qualitative and quantitative process methodologies that are well established in other fields of science such as anthropology and social sciences; this research can help clinicians determine the goodness of fit of these methodologies for gathering scientific evidence in the field of multicultural infant–family mental health.

At this juncture, it seems fitting that we end this chapter by reflecting on why this training and research process—with its focus on presence, connection, attunement, and competence—has been significant for us. As multicultural infant–family mental health clinicians, we acknowledge that babies take us back to the babies in ourselves. "They awaken in us a thirst that sleeps deep within some wellspring of yearning that we know we have neglected" (Schafer, 2004, p. 8). This yearning is for more than biological survival. It is a yearning for presence, openness, connectedness, fullness, and joy. In our endeavor to understand babies and to work with them and their early relationships, we have to let ourselves enter into their realm of centered presence, openness, curiosity, awareness, and joy. We cannot mimic or pretend to embody these elements, as babies do not pretend. In return for their authentic and genuine presence with us, we cannot be anything but authentic and genuine in our interactions with them.

Schafer (2004) says that in the process of growing up, we have veiled our spiritual selves and cloaked these selves with "psychological structures of so-called maturity" (p. 4) that have robbed us of our understanding of infancy and our natural capacity for holistic presence. In the Hindu philosophy, the human self is seen as the Infinite or the Absolute (known as "Aham Brahmasmi") that is, by nature, the same as another human self (Karuppaswamy & Natrajan, 2005). So, it is believed that the barriers between "you" and "I" (that inhibit presence) are an illusion that can be removed by deepening awareness and self-realization. Such meanings and experiences speak to the need for unveiling ourselves and becoming aware of our spiritual nature, which then can help us connect with the core of such experiences in infancy, a place in which we have all been. Our journey in our training process has been a process of becoming more aware of this place and owning our innate capacities to remember, understand, and be in the spiritual realms that infants can take us to as articulated by Schafer. These realms are those of genuine presence, joy, and awareness of other's awareness. Schafer articulated these three realms of experience in a very short, clear, and powerful paper in an effort to bring awareness to, and connect spiritual and human aspects of development for, multicultural infant–family mental health professionals.

References

Avis, J. M., & Sprenkle, D. H. (1990). Outcome research on family therapy training: A substantive and methodological review. *Journal of Marital & Family Therapy, 16,* 241–264.

Banerjee, L. (2000). Self-development practices for professionals: Gems from the family therapy field. *Psychological Foundations: The Journal, 11*(2), 48–54.

Banerjee, L. (2006, March). *Hearing the voices of infants, toddlers and preschoolers using Circles of Experience: A clinician's guide.* Paper presented at the First International Conference of the Indian Association of Family Therapy, New Delhi, India.

Banerjee, L., & Willingham, M. (1998). Self-awareness development. *Journal of Research and Applications in Clinical Psychology, 1*(2), 1–15.

Boszormenyi-Nagy, I., & Krasner, B. (1986). *Between give and take: A clinical guide to contextual therapy.* New York: Brunner/Mazel.

Bowen, M. (1985). *Family therapy in clinical practice.* Northvale, NJ: Jason Aronson.

Bugental, J. F. T. (1978). *Psychotherapy and process.* Menlo Park, NJ: Addison-Wesley.

Campbell, D., Bianco, V., Dowling, E., Goldberg, H., McNab, S., & Pentecost, D. (2003). Family therapy for childhood depression: Researching significant moments. *Journal of Family Therapy, 25,* 417–435.

Clark, A. (1979). On being centered. *Gestalt Journal, 2,* 35–49.

Csikszentmihalyi, M. (1990). *Flow: The psychology of optimal experience.* New York: Harper Perennial.

Deacon, T. (1997). *The symbolic species.* New York: W. W. Norton.

Geller, S. M. (2001). Therapists' presence: The development of a model and a measure (Doctoral dissertation, York University, 2001). *Dissertation Abstracts International, 63,* 1025.

Guba, E., & Lincoln, Y. (1994). Competing paradigms in qualitative research. In N. K. Denzin & Y. S. Lincoln (Eds.), *Handbook of qualitative research* (pp. 105–117). Thousand Oaks, CA: Sage.

Heffron, M. C. (2005). Reflective supervision in infant, toddler, and preschool work. In K. M. Finello (Ed.), *The handbook of training and practice in infant and preschool mental health* (pp. 114–136). San Francisco: Jossey-Bass.

Heppner, P., Kivlighan, D., & Wampold, B. (1999). *Research design in counseling.* San Francisco: Thomson Wadsworth.

Hill, C. E. (1982). Counseling process researcher: Philosophical and methodological dilemmas. *The Consulting Psychologist, 10*(4), 7–20.

Hycner, R. (1953). *Between person and person: Towards a dialogical psychotherapy.* New York: The Gestalt Journal Press.

Hycner, R., & Jacobs, L. (1995). *The healing relationship in gestalt therapy: A dialogical/self psychology approach.* New York: The Gestalt Journal Press.

Karuppaswamy, N., & Natrajan, R. (2005). Family therapy from a Hindu Indian worldview. In M. Rastogi & E. Wieling (Eds.), *Voices of color: First person accounts of ethnic minority therapists* (pp. 297–312). Thousand Oaks, CA: Sage.

Keefe, T. (1975). Meditation and the psychotherapist. *American Journal of Orthopsychiatry, 45,* 484–489.

Kempler, W. (1970). The therapists' merchandise. *Voices, 5,* 57–60.

Lambert, M. J., & Hill, C. E. (1994). Assessing psychotherapy outcomes and processes. In A. E. Bergins & S. L. Garfield (Eds.), *Handbook of psychotherapy and behavior change* (pp. 72–113). New York: Wiley.

Lawless, J., Gale, J., & Bacigalupe, G. (2001). The discourse of race and culture in family therapy supervision. *Contemporary Family Therapy, 23,* 181–197.

Lieberman, M. A., Yalom, I. D., & Miles, M. B. (1973). *Encounter groups: First facts.* New York: Basic Books.

Lietaer, G. (1993). Authenticity, congruence, and transparency. In D. Brazier (Ed.), *Beyond Carl Rogers: Toward a psychotherapy for the twenty-first century* (pp. 17–46). London: Constable and Company.

Maturana, H. R., & Varela, F. J. (1987). *The tree of knowledge.* Boston: New Science Library.

May, R. (1958). Contributions to existential therapy. In R. May, E. Angel, & H. Ellenberger (Eds.), *Existence: A new dimension in psychiatry and psychology* (pp. 37–91). New York: Basic Books.

McConnaughy, E. A. (1987). The person of the therapist in psychotherapeutic practice. *Psychotherapy, 24,* 303–314.

McDaniel, S., & Landau-Stanton, J. (1991). Family-of-origin work and family therapy skills training: Both-and. *Family Process, 30,* 459-471.

Mertens, D. M. (2005). *Research methods in education and psychology.* Thousand Oaks, CA: Sage.

Minuchin, P., Colapinto, J., & Minuchin, S. (1998). *Working with families of the poor.* New York: Guilford Press.

Minuchin, S. (1974). *Families and family therapy.* Cambridge, MA: Harvard University Press.

Minuchin, S., & Fishman, C. H. (1981). *Family therapy techniques.* Cambridge, MA: Harvard University Press.

Minuchin, S., Lee, W. Y., & Simon, G. M. (1996). *Mastering family therapy.* New York: Wiley.

Minuchin, S., & Nichols, M. (1993). *Family healing: Strategies for hope and understanding.* New York: Simon & Schuster.

Onunaku, N., Gilkerson, L., & Ahlers, T. (2006). Building a comprehensive mental health system for young children. *Zero to Three, 26,* 34–40.

Patterson, J., Williams, L., Grauf-Grounds, C., & Chamow, L. (1998). *Essential skills in family therapy: From the first interview to termination.* New York: Guilford Press.

Patton, M. (2002). *Qualitative research and evaluation methods* (3rd ed.). Thousand Oaks, CA: Sage.

Pinsof, W., & Wynne, L. (2000). Towards progress research: Closing the gap between family therapy practice and research. *Journal of Marital & Family Therapy, 26,* 1–8.

Polite, K., & Bourg, E. (1991). Relationship competency. In R. L. Peterson, J. D. McHolland, R. J. Bent, E. Davis-Russell, G. E. Edwall, K. Polite, et al. (Eds.), *The core curriculum in professional psychology* (pp. 83–88). Washington, DC: American Psychological Association.

Prochaska, J. O., & Prochaska, J. M. (1999). Why don't continents move? Why don't people change? *Journal of Psychotherapy Integration, 9,* 83–102.

Rogers, C. R. (1957). The necessary and sufficient conditions of therapeutic personality change. *Journal of Consulting Psychology, 21,* 97–103.

Rotenstreich, N. (1967). The right and the limitations of Buber's dialogical thought. In P. A. Schlipp & M. S. Friedman (Eds.), *The philosophy of Martin Buber.* (*The library of living philosophers,* Vol. 27; pp. 97–132). La Salle, Illinois: Cambridge University Press.

Sameroff, A. J., & Mackenzie, M. J. (2003). A quarter-century of the transactional model: How have things changed? *Zero to Three, 24,* 14–22.

Santorelli, S. (1999). *Heal thy self: Lessons on mindfulness in medicine.* New York: Bell Tower.

Satir, V. (1987). The therapist story. *Journal of Psychotherapy and the Family, 3,* 17–23.

Schafer, W. (2004). The infant as reflection of soul: The time before there was a self. *Zero to Three, 24,* 4–8.

Schur, T. J. (2002). Supervision as a disciplined focus on self and not the other: A different systems model. *Contemporary Family Therapy, 24,* 399–422.

Siegal, D. J. (1999). *The developing mind.* New York: Guilford Press.

Stern, D. (1995). *The motherhood constellation.* New York: Basic Books.

Street, E. (1997). Family therapy training research: An updating review. *Journal of Family Therapy, 19,* 89–111.

Street, E. (1988). Family therapy training research: System model and review. *Journal of Family Therapy, 10,* 383–402.

Thistle, P. (1981). The therapist's own family: Focus of training for family therapists. *Social Work, 26,* 248–250.

Timm, T. M., & Blow, A. J. (1999). Self-of-the-therapist work: A balance between removing restraints and identifying resources. *Contemporary Family Therapy, 21*(3), 331–351.

Tucker, S., & Pinsof, W. (1984). The empirical evaluation of structural family therapy training. *Family Process, 23,* 437–456.

Weatherston, D. J. (2005). Returning the treasure to babies: An introduction to infant mental health service and training. In K. M. Finello (Ed.), *The handbook of training and practice in infant and preschool mental health* (pp. 3–30). San Francisco: Jossey-Bass.

Williamson, D. (1981). Personal authority via termination of the intergenerational hierarchical boundary: A "new" stage in the family life cycle. *Journal of Marital & Family Therapy, 7,* 441–452.

Wolf, F. A. (1988). *Parallel universes: The search for other worlds.* New York: Simon & Schuster.

Wolfson, R. (2003). *Simply Einstein: Relativity demystified.* New York: W. W. Norton.

Yalom, I. D. (1995). *The theory and practice of group psychotherapy* (4th ed.). New York: Basic Books.

ZERO TO THREE. (2004). *Zero to Three fact sheet.* Washington, DC: Author.

EPILOGUE

CHAPTER 9

The Placental Ground of Experience—A Source of Connection, Meaning, and Presence: Paradigmatic Considerations

Leena Banerjee Brown

in bird leis
the birds were flying only they were birds from before
and from afterwards so that nobody could see them.
—William S. Merwin, 1998 (p. 20)

My research has shown me that when emotions are expressed, which is to say that the bio-chemicals that are the substrate of emotion are flowing freely, all systems are united and made whole . . . . the idea of the network is still too new to have affected the way mainstream medicine and psychology deal with our health and our illnesses.
—Candace B. Pert, 1997 (p. 273, 274)

Whether in poetry, as in the words of William S. Merwin, or in neuroscience, as in the words of Candace B. Pert, one of its pioneering researchers, the flow of experience across time and systems finds voice, as do its mysteries and clarities. *Circles* emphasizes the place of experience in professional endeavors as a place of placental significance in which awareness can arise and grow. Several things are meant by the term *experience*. First, it refers to being open, alive, joyful, engaged, and present in the moment in relationships and events as well as being fully present in the here and now. By its very nature, attending to experience shifts us into inclusive and integrative (dual emotional–cognitive) engagement with phenomena. This shift occurs because experience includes sensations, feelings, thoughts, and actions and is more than each of these parts because it integrates each of them with one another and with memory to create connection and meaning. By attending to experience, we expand our attention and awareness to include all of these inputs and become more aware of process, obvious and subtle, spoken and unspoken, tangible and intangible, concrete and symbolic. Through the inclusion and integration of these varied aspects of experience, we grasp the heart of a conversation or relationship, the climate and culture of a context, the spirit of a moment. Experiences register in our brains and in our bodies, change our brains and body through our electrophysiology and neurochemistry, and interact with our biochemistry. They register in our relationships through lessons lived, learned, and remembered, thus facilitating greater awareness, flexibility, and growth. Or they obstruct awareness through unresolved, unintegrated, traumatic experiences that manifest as rigidities and resistances. Experiences can be available for both inner reflection and learning as well as for both interpersonal reflection and collaborative learning. Reflective practices connect individuals and collectives to experiences of deeper states of self-understanding and empathy as well as compassion for oneself and others.

Experience is a container in which the subjective and objective domains of knowledge intersect and connect, and self-awareness development is one way of gaining deeper access into this container. The subjective aspect of experience is an up-close aspect of becoming in touch with the fullness of the experience in the moment. The objective aspect is a stepping-back aspect of engaging in inquiry, taking into account context, history, and available funds of information. The integration of the two parts returns us to the subjective with new insight, information, and meaning. Thus, the dance of the subjective and the objective elements in experience continues. This dance is beautifully depicted as the flow of energy and information (Siegal, 1999), which is a descriptor of reality at a core level that can be experienced and known. Energy, which is all pervasive, becomes information when it is organized into specific patterns (Simon, 2000). It flows within us in our brains and bodies; between us in our relationships; within computers and in the communications between them; and in other technological devices, on printed pages, in flowing rivers, in a baby's bathwater, and in the smiles, touch, and sounds exchanged among a baby and members of her family.

Developmental science has long established that human beings are unique in their ability to (a) build and guide their lives with a systematized set of meanings represented in beliefs and practices that we call *culture* and (b) use language and its symbols to communicate these meanings. The methodologies that we use to gain useful and applicable knowledge and strategies for our species—most especially, for the very young of our species—need to take into account meaning in all of the depth and breadth in which it is available to us in our experience. Thus, we must engage in sophisticated integrations of subjective and objective methodologies, moving beyond traditional science's notion of the supremacy of quantitative, objective methods of inquiry. We are living in times in which the theoretical formulations in physical science have far outpaced available scientific methodologies necessary for corroborating them. We are learning, from advances in the natural sciences, that we can be in two places at once, and that we can be two things at once, such as a wave and a particle. We are learning that atoms can spin clockwise and counterclockwise simultaneously and that matter larger than atoms can act in ways that challenge conventional notions of reality and fantasy, fact and fiction. Schafer (2004, p. 8), observing similar facts, calls for the field of infant studies to take the lead in "fashioning" a "new synthesis." Indeed, the beginning of life in the newborn and in the young child is a time that calls parents, families, and communities to new opportunities for new experiences that are synthesized into new awareness. It is entirely reasonable that knowledge bases and practices that are founded on an intact and integrated framework of spirit, mind, and body can feed this opportunity and awareness in a more full and satisfying way.

It is time for collaborative dialogue in the human sciences between subjective and objective routes to knowledge systematized into methodologies, especially those individuals involved in advancing the quality of human existence in the cradle of life. The goal of such dialogue is engaging in the development of an integrative paradigm constituted by subjective and objective methodologies, with art and traditionally defined science acting as equal partners in unraveling the mysteries of existence. Rachel Fulton (Gibson, 2006), an historian at the University of Chicago, speaks of the need for advancing and deepening understanding in her discipline through *scholarly empathy*, which is defined as the recognition of being a part of the interpretive circle, similar to being the observer or participant who perturbs and changes that which is studied. Fulton (Gibson, 2006) argues that such acknowledgment is frightening for historians and explains the preference for staying outside and for leaving out or bypassing deeper understandings. This critique is relevant across disciplines and, indeed, applies to august bodies of literature in the multicultural infant–family mental health field that await the integration of scholarly empathy. It awaits the day when researchers, scholars, practitioners, and policymakers will routinely connect with, acknowledge, and delve into the role of their subjective experiences and perspectives in the evidence that they produce, use, and advocate because there simply is no such thing as complete objectivity, nor, given the nature of things, is such a goal desirable.

The call, then, is for an integrative scientific paradigm generating methodologies with which we can inquire into phenomena. It is a call for dynamic and synchronous synthesis of multiple information sources gathered from subjective and objective domains, yielding highly informed, refined, and deep understandings. It opens up the possibility that the microcosm, subjectively seen, will unveil the macrocosm and that the macrocosm, objectively seen, will reveal the microcosm. Kabat-Zinn (2003, p. 145) describes the Buddha as a "born scientist and physician who had nothing in the way of instrumentation other than his own mind, body, and experience." He goes on to describe the Buddha's "arduous and single-minded contemplative investigations" (Kabat-Zinn, 2003, p. 145) and "deep, penetrative non-conceptual seeing into the nature of mind and world" (Kabat-Zinn, 2003, p. 146) that produced profound insights on human nature and medicine for its various states of imbalance and disease. Imagine our collective investment in an integrative scientific paradigm that holds open the possibility for such seeing, which may be described, using the words of William Blake, as "seeing the universe in a grain of sand and eternity in an hour."

The integrative paradigm immediately and routinely shifts the experience of hierarchy in relationships created by the hierarchical separation of the knowledge and expertise bearer and the recipient. The paradigm moves this experience to one of collaboration that puts the professional and the client on the same plane as human beings who have different roles. Such shifts in relationships, when they occur sustainably, are experiential and grow out of the culture of the training and work context. People experience the shift as movement from a fractured, hierarchical paradigm—in which spirit and the experience of phenomena are left out and the intellect is put above all else—to an integrated paradigm—in which one accepts all aspects of reality in a curious, even, and equal way, seeking to learn and grow through experience in a journey without end. This integrated paradigm shifts from a rhetoric of collaboration between client and professional, clinician and researcher, field workers and policymakers, to the actual, authentic experience of collaboration.

Experience is the container in which the infant lives. Long before an infant can speak, she can experience the world through sense perceptions, movement, and emotional states. She can relate to caregivers by expressing her need for nourishment, warmth, comfort, and security. She can express a range of feelings, from contentment to distress. She has psychological needs for being empathically seen, heard, and responded to. Her experience of her caregivers' responsivity to these needs and feelings, as well as their provision of care and protection, contributes to her early, implicit memories and sense of self (Siegal, 1999). She registers her experiences in her emotional brain as the neocortex is still in the early stages of development. She also embodies her experiences in the vertical neural network that runs through her body, with the networks in the heart and the gut being, perhaps, especially pertinent (Siegal, 2006). These implicit memories carry her early experiences of herself and her world.

As language emerges in toddlerhood, she begins to accumulate explicit or conscious memories, but she may continue to enact implicit memories through participatory memories (Fogel, 2004), pointing to the close and integral early connections between perceptual and motor development. Research provides ample evidence that each infant and young child's early experiences of perception and movement, alone, are highly individual (Greenspan, 1993). Therefore, a professional can be adequately prepared to access, connect, and work in multicultural infant mental health if integration of current objective knowledge with subjective experience facilitates deep, empathic understanding of the individuality of each child.

Objective inquiry has flourished in recent centuries, and its methodologies have been developed and are being continually refined. The discipline and methods of work necessary for deep subjective connection to phenomena in professional work have suffered pervasive neglect and deprivation. Reflective process, stories/narratives, self-awareness and self-care processes, qualitative inquiry, contemplative process, and meditation are merely some methods of subjective inquiry that are in their infancy in the modern professional arena. However, these methods rest on long histories of development in many cultures around the globe, and they call to pioneers who can bring them to light in relevant ways for current use in the global nursery and for all of those individuals dedicated to serving it.

Meditation itself is a "highly refined practice aimed at systematically training and cultivating various aspects of mind and heart via the faculty of mindful attention" (Kabat-Zinn, 2003, p. 145) that includes the attitudes of openness, receptivity, warmth, and compassion. Imagine a national institute of wellness that is dedicated to such work, and imagine the multicultural infant–family mental health field at the forefront. Imagine the development of a national network of mentors and role models who contribute to the creation of an integrative paradigm and inspire others to engage and contribute. Imagine the organization of a seminal series of national and international conferences dedicated to formative dialogue on an integrative paradigm for knowledge and practice.

> *He alone*
> *who is joined to the horizon*
> *Can build new roads.*
> —Adonis (translated from Arabic by Khaled Mattawa, 2006)

This call for a paradigmatic shift to an integrative paradigm is a call to search for ideas, strategies, practices, and methodologies that can guide actual shifts in thinking, practice, research, and policy. It is a call to transform and expand our epistemologies, paradigms of knowledge, and institutional cultures to grow beyond the limitations of an old and imbalanced paradigm and to be open and facilitative of new complexities in an integrative paradigm. It is a call to connect deeply with the placental ground of experience as inspiration and guide in this process. If Bronfenbrenner's (1979) Circles were a call for context and breadth in the multicultural infant–family field, these Circles are a call for depth, complexity, and integration. In the poet's words, this call reads as follows:

> *The same stream of life that runs through my veins runs through the world, and dances in rhythmic measure. It is the same life that shoots through numberless blades of grass and breaks into tumultuous waves of leaves and flowers. It is the same life that is rocked in the ocean cradle of life and death in ebb and in flow. I feel my limbs are made glorious by the touch of this world of life and my pride is*

from the life throb of ages dancing in my blood this moment.
—Rabindranath Tagore, Nobel Laureate in Literature, 1913 (as cited in Chopra, 1990)

References

Adonis. (2006). *Childhood* (K. Mattawa, Trans.). Retrieved January 1, 2007, from www.deviantart.com/deviation/33885205

Bronfenbrenner, U. (1979). *The ecology of human development: Experiments by nature and design.* Cambridge, MA: Harvard University Press.

Chopra, D. (1990). *The new physics of healing: Inside the medicine of the future.* Boulder, CO: Sounds True Recordings.

Fogel, A. (2004). Remembering infancy: Accessing our earliest experiences. In G. Bremner & A. Slater (Eds.), *Theories of infant development* (pp. 204–230). Cambridge, England: Blackwell.

Gibson, L. (2006). Mirrored emotion. *University of Chicago Magazine, 98*(4), 34–39.

Greenspan, S. (1993). *Playground politics: Understanding the emotional life of your school-age child.* Reading, MA: Perseus Books.

Kabat-Zinn, J. (2003). Mindfulness-based interventions in context: Past, present and future. *Clinical Psychology: Science and Practice, 10*(2), 144–156.

Merwin, W. S. (1998). *The folding cliffs: A narrative of 19th-century Hawaii.* New York: Alfred A. Knopf.

Pert, C. B. (1997). *The molecules of emotion: The science behind mind–body medicine.* New York: Scribner.

Schafer, W. (2004). The infant as reflection of soul: The time before there was a self. *Zero to Three, 24,* 4–8.

Siegal, D. J. (1999). *The developing mind.* New York: Guilford Press.

Siegal, D. J. (2006, March). *Awakening the mind to the wisdom of the body.* Paper presented at The Embodied Mind: Integration of the Body, Brain, and Mind in Clinical Practice: A UCLA Extension and Lifespan Learning Institute Conference, Los Angeles.

Simon, D. (2000). *Return to wholeness: Embracing body, mind, and spirit in the face of cancer.* New York: Wiley.

ABOUT THE AUTHORS

Leena Banerjee Brown, PhD, is professor of clinical psychology at Alliant International University's California School of Professional Psychology, Los Angeles, where she has been training doctoral students for seventeen years. She has three children of her own. She was instrumental in starting Mother Infant Support Team in Hawaii, a tertiary child abuse prevention program that works with Healthy Start programs. More recently, she helped to start Early Connections, an outpatient community mental health program that serves infants, toddlers, young children, and their families in Los Angeles County, California.

Michael Barrazza, MA, is a doctoral candidate at Alliant International University's California School of Professional Psychology, Los Angeles. His emphasis is on multicultural community clinical psychology.

Tasha Boucher, MA, MFT, is a child–family clinician who focuses on providing home- and center-based mental health services to families with young children. She serves in this role at Early Connections at Bienvenidos Children's Center, Inc., in Montebello, CA.

Matthew Calkins, PsyD, is the Manager of Early Connections, a multisite mental health program serving families with children age birth to 5 at Bienvenidos Children's Center, Inc. He also maintains a private practice in psychotherapy in South Pasadena, CA.

Lucia Lopez-Plunkett, PhD, is coordinator of Early Connections at Bienvenidos Children's Center, Inc., in Pomona, CA. She is bilingual and has substantial clinical experience with infants, toddlers, and their families. She also has an infant and a toddler of her own. She is dedicated to providing multiculturally competent, home-based services to vulnerable newborns, toddlers, and their families.

Raji Natrajan, PhD, is assistant professor of marriage and family therapy at Alliant International University. She serves as participant–researcher for the Early Connections program at Bienvenidos Children's Center, Inc., and has a newborn of her own.

Brooke Nisen, MA, MFT, is a child–family clinician at Early Connections at Bienvenidos Children's Center, Inc., in Altadena, CA. She is also the coordinator of the Multidisciplinary Assessment Team at Bienvenidos Children's Center, Inc. She has extensive experience working with young children in foster care.

Patricia Rosas, MSW, is a child–family clinician at Early Connections at Bienvenidos Children's Center, Inc., in Altadena, CA. She has worked with young children and families in residential and outpatient mental health settings, as well as with foster care and Head Start populations.